when
food
is a four-letter word

programs for recovery from anorexia, bulimia, bulimarexia, obesity, and other appetite disorders

Paul Haskew and Cynthia H. Adams

A SPECTRUM BOOK

Prentice-Hall, Inc., Englewood Cliffs, New Jersey 07632

Library of Congress Cataloging in Publication Data

Haskew, Paul.
    When food is a four-letter word.

    "A Spectrum Book."
    Bibliography: p.
    Includes index.
    I. Appetite disorders.   I. Adams, Cynthia H.
(date)   II. Title   III. Title: When food is a
4-letter word.
RC552.A72H37 1984   616.3'9   83-24520
ISBN 0-13-956111-0
ISBN 0-13-956103-X (pbk.)

10 9 8 7 6 5 4 3 2 1

ISBN 0-13-956111-0

ISBN 0-13-956103-X {PBK.}

Editorial/production supervision by Norma G. Ledbetter
Cover design © 1984 by Jeannette Jacobs
Manufacturing buyer: Doreen Cavallo

PRENTICE-HALL INTERNATIONAL, INC., *London*
PRENTICE-HALL OF AUSTRALIA PTY. LIMITED, *Sydney*
PRENTICE-HALL CANADA INC., *Toronto*
PRENTICE-HALL OF INDIA PRIVATE LIMITED, *New Delhi*
PRENTICE-HALL OF JAPAN, INC., *Tokyo*
PRENTICE-HALL OF SOUTHEAST ASIA PTE. LTD., *Singapore*
WHITEHALL BOOKS LIMITED, *Wellington, New Zealand*
EDITORA PRENTICE-HALL DO BRASIL LTDA., *Rio de Janeiro*

to our spouses,
Irene and Roger,
and our children,
Derek, Penelope, and Andrew,
with love

contents

preface

Have you heard or read about terms such as *anorexia* and *bulimia*? Do these words make you think of some rare illness suffered by some unlucky few? If so, you are wrong.

Have you gone through periods of being concerned, almost to the point of obsession, about your weight? Do you feel ashamed of every ounce of fat on your body? Have you tried a number of different diet programs? If so, this book is for you.

A peculiar obsession has arisen in Western society. A fear of fat and a desire to be thin have overcome rational thought in the minds of millions. The consequences of our obsession with thinness are needless misery for many. And, as always happens when people want what they cannot have, it has handsomely enriched opportunists who trade on such fads and fears.

Fashion has declared that gaunt and bony is beautiful. Medicine has declared (with inappropriate firmness and insufficient hard facts) that obesity is hazardous to our health. Women have found that a feminine fullness handicaps their struggle to compete as equals with men. The postwar baby boom has reached middle age and begun to experience "middle-aged spread."

Upset because we no longer feel or look twenty-five, millions of us have taken up the battle against fat. Meanwhile, the food industry has learned to employ the most persuasive advertising techniques to market low-quality, high-profit, high-calorie manufactured foods to a populace that has less time and less opportunity to prepare nutritious meals from unprocessed foodstuffs.

Finally, and perhaps most important of all, there is a widespread illusion that the concept of all men being created equal means that everyone, but especially every woman, has an equal opportunity and an equal responsibility to fit the current norms for acceptable appearance. To assert that not everyone can or should be thin may be to risk being labeled sexist or undemocratic, but that's exactly what we're doing.

The impact of powerful social pressures on young people to be thin has been predictably calamitous. Children in grade school can be heard chatting with one another about the latest fad diet. With innocent daring and a sincere desire to fit in, they begin battle with their appetites in an unwitting attempt to stem their normal development. In our high schools today, anorexia is rampant, and self-starvation has come to be a common expression of strength and status. Even punitive and self-abusive exercising is perceived as a minimal response to the need to avoid getting fat.

Adults, too, with barely greater sophistication, furiously diet, exercise, and medicate themselves in a struggle to achieve or maintain a thin figure.

Few, if any, of these people realize that in resolving to reduce their widths, they are taking on adversaries of formidable strength—namely, their own minds and bodies. Some will succeed in "disciplining" themselves. Others will come to recognize that they are losing the battle and seek a compromise. Many will engage in periodic battles with fat, using books and programs that help them lose a few pounds now and then, only to gain them back a month or two later. The rest will become casualties: victims to greater or lesser degrees of compulsive eating, bulimia, anorexia, self-induced vomiting, laxative abuse, anxiety, depression, isolation, self-hatred, and weight gain.

Our purpose is to present, in a concise and readable format, enough details about this epidemic of appetite disorders to enable informed persons, concerned parents, educators, and health professionals to understand, relieve, and even prevent them. In one volume we address both eating disorders and obesity, which we see as separate but related topics.

This book presents the knowledge we have gained through the work of others, through our own research, and most important, through the lessons our students have taught us. Although the examples that we present are fictional, so that confidentiality is preserved, they are all based on behaviors we have observed and statements we have heard. They provide an insider's view of the harsh struggles, and sometimes remarkable outcomes, of our work with a small part of a national epidemic.

Our own clinical experience and the research literature have convinced us that our approach is psychologically and physiologically sound, that it provides appetite-disordered persons with new ways of thinking and acting that allow them to regain their health, strength, and self-respect.

In preparing this book, we have been greatly helped by the support and encouragement of our colleagues in the University Health Service and School of Allied Health Professions at the University of Connecticut, most especially Dr. Joe Nowinski and Dean Polly Fitz. Our greatest debt of gratitude, however, is owed to the many clients and students whose insights pointed the ways to recovery and helped form the ideas that have in turn enabled us to help others.

1

appetite disorder
the dieter's disease

―――――――――――――――――――――

*"It's not that I want to be one of the crowd,
but I do want to be what the crowd thinks is best."*

The quest for beauty surely began at the dawn of society, and the search for relief from unfashionable fatness may be almost as old. The Romans' use of vomitoriums and the Victorians' inclusion of live tape worms in their diet are two of the more bizarre, though probably more successful, techniques that have been employed in that pursuit. A third technique—dieting—has also always been known and used.

Penny always knew she was fat; however, her weight wasn't always a problem. When her preschool ballet teacher, for example, assigned her to the second row in the chorus and gave her the lead in "The Teddy Bears Picnic," she was content in the belief that there is a place in the sun for everyone. In grade school, she enjoyed being the first in her class to fit into grown-up clothes. In junior high, when her bust filled quickly to splendid dimensions, she felt mature and female. In those years, being fat was not a disability.

At fifteen, Penny's world fell apart. Overnight, it seemed, she had become everything nobody wanted to be. The phone stopped ringing, her friends paired off without her, and she began to feel like a leper.

Penny's mother knew what had happened; so did her dad. Fat people themselves, they had known rejection too, but though they ached to be of help, Penny's eyes blazed with blame and disgust whenever they tried to talk to her. They watched helplessly as she withdrew and started to diet.

Because dieting is undoubtedly successful in causing an initial weight loss, any reluctance to diet counts heavily against fat people in public opinion. In addition, the assumption that obesity is the result of gluttony and a lack of self-control has created an almost universal suspicion that obesity must be the visible sign of a poor or weak character. This view is rarely stated so bluntly, but it does not have to be. Instead, a cultural prejudice against overweight people says it silently and with a devastating effect on its victims. Think of the word FAT. What kind of associations do you have?

This prejudice against people who are fat is possibly the single greatest cause of self-hatred in our culture. It is a self-hatred that breeds an endless variety of other emotional disorders and that feeds a multibillion dollar industry dedicated to providing salves and quick-but-false solutions to tens of millions of unhappy people. It is a self-hatred that is wholly undeserved.

From experimental data, scientists studying the causes of obesity have developed a few theories, a few conclusions, and many unanswered questions. One thing that is clear is that people who are statistically overweight are no more or less guilty of poor or weak character than anyone else. Some are simply big people: men and women who are born programmed to develop large fat deposits and who therefore are naturally heavy. Others have a tendency to store energy as fat when they fail to match their food intake to their energy needs, and, as a result, they experience major increases in weight. This is in contrast to people who maintain a consistent weight, who also eat more than they need, but whose bodies use other means to dispose of the excess.

A tendency towards being overweight and being obese might be regarded as an illness or disability only to the extent that it impairs health and shortens life: a circumstance that may be rarer than is generally supposed. Unfortunately, many healthy but large people are less concerned about their lifespan than the impact of their size and shape on their social life and self-esteem. Too often their reaction to the unremitting discrimination they experience is to seek cosmetic changes in their appearance through endless varieties of malnutrition that they prefer to think of as "dieting."

Paradoxically and tragically, for many people the net effect of their attempts to lose weight is to further aggravate their bodies' tendency to store fat. Worse, in the process they often sharpen their appetites, so that excess eating becomes even more likely. It is these side effects of dieting and being overweight that this book is principally concerned with—side effects that have immense social, psychological, and physical consequences for people who suffer from them. They constitute a syndrome of disorders that includes anorexia, bulimia, bulimarexia, and compulsive eating.

All these aberrations have the distressing effect of alienating people from one of life's chief pleasures—eating—and of making an enemy of a healthy natural attribute: appetite. It has become customary to refer to them as *eating disorders*, and they are clearly that. At a more fundamental level, though, the struggle is with *appetite*. It is not the act of eating that has become disordered but the *urge* to eat that cannot be properly regulated. This gives rise to the extreme behaviors of self-starvation on the one hand and outrageous bingeing on the other. The bingeing, in turn, may instigate compensatory measures such as deliberate vomiting or purging.

For these reasons, we have coined the term *pathorexia*, meaning "disordered appetite," to refer to the whole spectrum of appetite and eating disorders. Pathorexia is a general term that incorporates anorexia, bulimia, bulimarexia, and other psychosomatic disorders of eating and appetite. It is not the first general term that has been used in this connection. In the 1960s, the word *dysorexia* was proposed, and later *dietary chaos syndrome* was used. These are terms that may have applied to someone in your family.

What we want to convey by using a general term such as *pathorexia* is the close relationship and interchangeability frequently seen among eating disorders. A helpful concept for forming an understanding of pathorexia comes from considering the difference between appetite and hunger. *Appetite* describes an emotional and physical impulse to eat, regardless of nutritional needs. *Hunger*, in contrast, refers to a physical urge to eat that is prompted by an immediate dietary deficiency.

In healthy people, hunger and appetite usually coincide. The occasions when they do not coincide include opportunites to eat treats and exotic offerings that arouse appetite even when we are not hungry. In another vein, traumatic events can be so unsettling that appetite is lost even though hunger pain and the need for food are present.

When pathorexia develops, the relationship between the desire to eat and the body's need for food is so discrepant that normal, healthy eating becomes the exception rather than the rule. This book is about those discrepancies, their causes, and their relationship to dieting, to being overweight, and to obesity. It is also a guide to their prevention and cure.

There is a distinct and crucial difference between *pathorexic* persons and fat people who do not overeat but who are simply naturally heavy. The range of naturally healthy human shapes is far greater than fashion dictates, and many (perhaps most) soft, round people are content with their lives, their appetites, and their bodies.

In Chapter 3, we deal specifically with problems related to obesity. Chapters 10 and 11 include some psychologically safe programs that can be used for weight loss. But we are primarily addressing *eating* and *appetite* disorders, not weight itself. The principal goal of this book is to help you distinguish between problems of eating, appetite, and weight, and to understand their relationship to each other. Our focus, too, is on those forms of pathorexia that are not so severe that they require hospitalization.

Much of what has been written to date on eating disorders has concentrated on the life threatening extreme of *anorexia nervosa*. We will not ignore this disturbing illness, but both our clinical work and this book deal mostly with the concerns of people whose appetite disorders, though painful and handicapping, are not so severe as to separate them from their families and friends. We want to promote understanding and provide relief for those millions of people whose struggle with physical, familial, and social pressures has caused them to lose touch with their appetites and has set them in conflict with their own bodies.

2
from diet to disaster
varieties of appetite disorder

> "I get so embarrassed about eating that when I do it,
> it feels like I'm having sex in public."

We have identified six ways in which people experience appetite disorders or pathorexia. They are: simple overeating, simple anorexia, anorexia nervosa, bulimia, bulimarexia, and oral expulsion. In this chapter we will discuss each one in that order. At the end there is a questionnaire that will help you rate your own degree of pathorexia.

There is considerable disagreement among experts about the names and definitions that we need to describe appetite disorders. Some prefer to regard all appetite disorders as varieties of anorexia nervosa. Others do not distinguish between bulimia and bulimarexia. Some writers refer to "anorexic-like behavior," the "binge-purge syndrome," and "bulimia nervosa." There is even less agreement about what overeating is. Pathorexia, is our way of simplifying the matter. All these other terms are varieties of pathorexia.

Simple Overeating

"Every time something goes wrong I want to eat, and every time something goes right I want to eat! When am I ever going to stop eating?"

Simple overeating is by far the commonest form of eating disorder, and is the way people respond to the loss of their natural ability to match their food intake with their energy output. For overeaters, the desire to eat almost always exceeds their need for food, so they either diet in an attempt to lose weight, or they allow their appetite free rein and store excess calories as fat.

We explain in Chapters 8 and 9 how a variety of physical and psychological factors operate to encourage eating and inhibit restraint, making overeaters more sensitive to some environmental cues that trigger eating.

Because our culture abounds in cues inviting us to eat, many overeaters are able to avoid excess intake only by adopting special controls, such as diets, calorie counting, or behavior modification programs that temporarily enable them to shut out the temptations to which they fall victim.

> A woman in her early forties, who had always been classified as obese, told us of a life made miserable by her weakness for eating. She began every day with a resolution to eat only three balanced meals, but she rarely got beyond ten o'clock in the morning without being seduced by something tasty. By evening, all semblance of her resolve was gone, and she would make a stop at the refrigerator or the pantry each time she moved around the house.

Overeaters resist focusing their attention on their appetite, even though they are well aware of the problems it creates for them. They worry instead about their bodies that they see as disfigured with excess fat. They look constantly for a simple and easy cure that will cause it to melt away.

Most overeaters experiment with appetite suppressing medications of some kind—over-the-counter, or prescription. In doing so, they acknowledge that it is their urge to eat that is the problem, but they rarely grasp the full importance of that concept. Instead, they think only of losing weight and view the pills as a means to that end, not as a way to experience living without the desire to overeat.

Simple overeaters are usually very unhappy about their behavior patterns but mask their feelings with a facade of good humor. They often make jokes about their weight or the way they eat. Underneath, however, they worry chronically about their appearance. Some overeaters monitor every person they meet, or even every person they catch sight of, and rank them all on a scale of thin to fat. In this way they keep track of their own place in a dismal and phony hierarchy.

Overeaters adopt many tricks to help them deny or conceal their weight, and their undisciplined eating. But every device of dress or posture and every public display of self-denial that is followed by secret eating, serves to increase their sense of isolation and chips away at their self-esteem. Sharing their weakness with fellow sufferers is a great tension reliever, so groups such as TOPS, Weight Watchers, and especially Overeaters Anonymous, provide them with valuable boosts in self-respect.

Simple Anorexia

"Really, I'd rather DIE than gain a single pound! I mean it! I mean it!"

Simple anorexia is a severe and unhealthy restriction of eating. Even though victims experience no loss of appetite they reject most opportunities to eat, and lose as much as one fifth of their normal weight. Most simple anorexics often appear to be on the verge of starvation; but some, whose normal figures are a bit rounded, manage to look very fashionable.

Even though their stated reason for losing weight is cosmetic, those who look physically too frail to be attractive, with hollow cheeks, thinning hair, and dark circles under their eyes, remain determined not to regain weight. They cannot see themselves as thin. Intensely afraid of being overweight and obese, they prefer to be skeletal rather than soft-textured and regard even their vestigial fat with distaste.

While often feeling faint and suffering other symptoms of malnutrition, they are surprisingly resilient and cope effectively with most aspects of everyday life.

> Anna was 68 pounds when we met her for the first time. At five feet two inches, she seemed desperately gaunt to us. Nevertheless, she was maintaining a full schedule of high-school activities, doing well academically, and keeping a place on the cheerleading squad. When she passed out at a practice one afternoon, the coach urged her to get a physical examination, but Anna rallied and talked her way out of taking action.
>
> Only when she passed out for the third time was she taken to the school nurse. Anna resisted every attempt to get her into treatment until she was forced to choose between seeing a therapist or being dropped as a cheerleader.

Many anorexics impose extra burdens upon themselves. They undertake rigorous regimens of running, swimming, situps, or dancing—not to improve physical fitness, but in pursuit of further weight loss. They survive for the duration of the disease—often many years—on diets that defy the basic principles of sound nutrition.

Anorexics are generally resistant to the most earnest and sincere efforts of their families and therapists who urge them to eat reasonable meals or set weight goals for them to work toward. This defiance has led many observers to conclude that family conflicts provoke much anorexic behavior. Indeed, family counseling often helps parents, brothers, and sisters avoid attitudes that promote or reinforce the self-starvation.

But it is clear, too, that many anorexics are primarily interested in pursuing thinness because they are convinced that it improves their appearance. And they get plenty of support for this view. They are often complimented on how well they wear clothes, they have no trouble getting dates, and they are envied by friends and acquaintances for their slimness and self discipline.

Anorexia may be a misnomer for this variety of pathorexia—it means *without appetite*—but anorexics are often consumed with thoughts of food. They may spend hours preparing meals for other people and are almost always ready to get into discussions about restaurants or recipes. Typically, too, from time to time they indulge in binges, often eating large amounts of rather unappetizing food such as bread, peanut butter, or cottage cheese.

They also hoard food in drawers and wardrobes, and then eat secretly, later throwing up what they have consumed. So it seems that appetite is more suppressed than lost, though after long periods without eating it may be much reduced.

There are indications that some anorexics may be responding to a minor brain dysfunction. This suggests the possibility that they may be physically predisposed to the disorder, and when they are experiencing the stresses that come with adolescence, they instinctively begin to starve themselves.

Anorexia is often the first type of pathorexia to be observed in a patient. Because of the metabolic changes caused by the fasting and because eating remains a troubling behavior even after recovery, anorexics may subsequently develop other forms of appetite disorder.

Many anorexics "know" that they are caught in a self-deluding web. Debbie, a high-school sophomore, told us about hers.

"Intellectually I didn't think that if I lost weight my problems would go away, but at another level I did. Every time I tricked my folks into thinking I'd had a meal but I hadn't, I felt strong and in control. It was the same when I weighed myself and I was lighter. . . . I stopped looking at the numbers after a while, they scared me, all I cared about was that I was just a bit less each time."

Debbie described how at times she would become more realistic, but that caused trouble too. "If I lost a whole pound I'd say to myself this is ridiculous, you've got to stop this, you know what you're doing to yourself! and I'd go have a snack. But it never ended there. I'd raid the refrigerator, then the pantry. Then I'd just keep eating because I'd know I was going to throw up. It was awful."

Despite their handicap, anorexics are usually very courteous in social and, initially at least, therapeutic contacts. These facades—polite, calm, agreeable, and hardworking—provide only poor mechanisms for dealing with anxiety, envy, disappointment, or aggression.

Anorexics are ill-equipped for adolescence and adulthood, where more competition, harsher skills and thicker skins are required. Confused about meeting these challenges, they pull back from growing up, turn anger inward, and seek control of unwelcome emotions through self-starvation. "I was so angry I could have lost twenty pounds!" expresses a common sentiment.

Such passive-agressive behavior confounds their parents, about whom the anorexics feel more intensely ambivalent than do normal adolescents.

Once the disorder is identified, a battle-royal may develop within the family, with parents pulled in many directions in their attempts to restore a traditional structure and order while their anorexic teenager typically explains that being left alone is all the help needed.

By making the body the focus of conflict with the parents, a teenager gains immense power and influence, as for all practical purposes, only that person decides whether or not to eat. But the struggle is always more complex than the anorexic person anticipates; family patterns of behavior do not change quickly, and the body has resources of its own to counteract the dangers of starvation so that the control that is perceived in dieting is often lost when the appetite overcomes willpower and a binge occurs.

Anorexia victims are at odds with society, using their bodies as weapons, but they find their bodies rebel against them too. It is hard to imagine the loneliness they feel when this happens, but their typical response is to redouble the effort to conquer their appetites rather than accept defeat. They bitterly resist the need for adequate restoration, and they refuse to seek comfort and support from loved ones.

Anorexia Nervosa

"Of course I'm still fat! Look at this, and this, and this! It's fat!"

Anorexia nervosa is simple anorexia carried to the point of insanity. The woman quoted above was five feet tall and weighed fifty-six pounds when she argued with her therapist about her condition.

In this stage of self-starvation, the appetite is truly lost, and body weight is at least twenty-five percent below normal. Victims lose all sense of reality with regard to food intake and, believing that they have conquered the need to eat, may literally starve to death. This may be the most lethal of the psychiatric disorders.

Persons suffering from anorexia nervosa require hospitalization and intensive medical and psychiatric intervention. Even then they remain in grave danger.

Identifying the line dividing simple anorexia, which is best treated on an out-patient basis, from anorexia nervosa, which is not, is a matter for careful professional judgment. Apart from substantial weight loss and associated physical problems, other considerations, such as the age of the patient, the degree of family discord, and the willingness to accept hospitalization, must be assessed.

Severe anorexics almost invariably resent intrusion by family and physicians. They frequently attempt to hide their weight loss by wearing bulky clothing. When not closely supervised, they sometimes conceal heavy objects in their pockets or drink large quantities of water prior to being weighed. When fed against their will, they often vomit their meals to prevent weight gain.

A nurse used the term "twilight zone" to describe the tragedy of losing a patient in intensive care to starvation.

"Chrissy was as nice a person as you could meet if you just wanted to talk. But as soon as nutrition in any form was proposed, she turned cold as ice. As far as she was concerned, we were assassinating her with our equipment, so she had a right to be angry. She said to me once, 'Starving keeps me sane.'"

Chrissy sabotaged every attempt that was made to get food into her. "The day before she died she was so weak she could barely move, but she still managed to put a crimp in her intravenous tube to stop it working, and then figured out how to disconnect the alarm. So it was an hour before we realized what she'd done. . . . When we were cleaning her room afterwards, we found two boxes of laxatives taped to the underside of the shelf in her cabinet.''

It has often been noted that anorexia nervosa is seen primarily in wealthy, high-status families. As recently as 1980, Gloria Leon, a prominent authority on eating disorders, reported that she had never seen a black anorexic. Today, however, we see persons of all ages, both sexes, and every social class becoming caught up in weight phobia, punitive dieting, and appetite disorder—though young people from wealthy professional families still predominate in clinic caseloads.

Severely impaired anorexics may suffer from a wide range of associated disabilities. They have a very poor understanding of their physical and emotional states. Body size and shape, for example, is a matter of great confusion for many who believe they are far larger and fatter than is the case. They often have lost the ability to recognize hunger or satiety, and sometimes this confusion extends to their emotions: patients may not know whether they are sad, angry, or even pleased, and may ask a parent or therapist to interpret their mood for them.

These distortions and deficits leave anorexics with little sense of control or trust. By focusing their entire attention on food, eating, exercise, and weight loss, they create the self-illusion of appropriate behavior while effectively isolating themselves from the corrective feedback and evaluations of their peers and family.

Left alone, they may become lethally turned in on themselves. Yet they have a terrible fear of having their insane world invaded. Only caring therapists and an awakened family can lead them back to the real world.

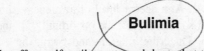

Bulimia

"I stuff myself until my stomach hurts, but that just slows me down. I don't quit until the food's all gone."

Also known as *hyperphagia,* bulimia is a variety of pathorexia characterized by episodes of voracious eating. On these occasions, outrageous bingeing may be indulged, during which anything and everything edible is stuffed in the mouth. The binges often end only when all available food has been consumed or when the victim's stomach is so filled that further eating becomes impossible. While bingeing, bulimics often feel peacefully removed from reality. Afterwards, they often feel intense remorse, and vow to them-selves that it will never happen again. But the promise is rarely kept for long. The major reason for bulimia is that victims simply give up the fight to control a seemingly insatiable desire to eat, and allow their appetite unrestrained expression.

> Many of our clients could identify with the woman who told us, "During the fat times in my life I had to force myself to go to work. Then I would rush home, pull the shades, unhook the phone, and sit on the floor next to the refrigerator eating myself into a stupor."

Typically, bulimics feel very guilty about their behavior. This causes them to be secretive about eating. When this is not possible in family settings, young bulimics may attempt to manipulate their parents into both curbing and per-mitting their overeating. An example of this was a child who requested that a lock be put on the refrigerator and that she be provided with a key!

Bulimics are just as anxious about weight and fat as other pathorexics, and their massive binges usually provoke substantial gains. The conflict between their craving to eat and their fear of obesity is often reduced by planning for binges, by fasting or limiting intake to low calories snacks, tea, or diet soda for several days.

Many bulimics find that a pattern of weekend indulgence preceeded and followed by weekday frugality is most easily sustained. Some binge only once a month, saving both money and calories, such that the overeating, once begun, can be of monumental proportions.

A common variety of bulimia requires the hyperphagia to be triggered off by a small surprise or upset. A party or holiday, or a rejection by a friend or other negative experience will do. Outside influence can then be blamed for the loss of control that follows. At a deeper level of awareness, the bulimic person knows, of course, that sooner or later the opportunity for indulgence will occur and will be taken. Once the binge is underway, the excuse for beginning it is forgotten.

Often the search for food becomes an obsession. Sometimes civilized behavior is abandoned if the only way to get food is through threats or theft.

> "One evening when I was totally out of control and there was nothing in the house, I raided garbage cans outside the apartments. I found a piece of watermelon and started to eat it when a guy came by with a bag of garbage. He looked at me strange, but he didn't know what I was doing, and, when he'd gone, I just kept on eating. It was after that night that I realized that I needed help."

Normal eaters also binge occasionally, and simple overeaters often report bingeing behaviors. Inquiry usually reveals these episodes as relatively minor when compared to the enormous intake of a true bulimic. A hyperphagic binge may consist of several pounds of food, perhaps as much or more than a family of four would consume in a day. Doughnuts by the dozen, ice cream by the carton, bread by the loaf, and peanut butter by the jar are the measures of quantity for the established bulimic.

Older and wealthier bulimics sometimes regulate and excuse their disorder by eating out. It is easier to justify a binge if someone else has a hand in its preparation. In *all you can eat* restaurants, their behavior can even be considered as having the endorsement of the management! From time to time, there are reports in the press of customers in these restaurants becoming so full that they collapse and die.

Bulimarexia

"At first I used to throw up to compensate for bingeing, but then I
realized I was only bingeing so that I could throw up."

As its name implies, this disorder is a combination of bulimic and anorexic behaviors. Bingeing is followed by purging with laxatives or self-induced vomiting. The cycle of binge-and-purge may be regularly spaced—a week or so apart—or it may be sporadic and unpredictable. Some victims are driven to frequent minor binges, such as eating a box of cookies and then quickly throwing up. This latter behavior may be repeated as often as twenty times a day taking the place of normal meals.

The term was coined by a psychologist at Cornell University, Marlene Boskind-White, who discovered that scores of women students were bingeing and purging. In her view, bulimarexia is a *learned* behavior that can be abondoned by learning better behaviors, backed by healthier attitudes about oneself. We agree with her, but in our experience many bulimarexics become enmeshed in physical and psychological complications resulting from the behavior that limit their freedom to give it up. For this reason, we believe that bulimarexia is not just a behavior. It is a disease.

Bulimarexia may be viewed as an extreme version of the simple overeater's pattern of excess eating followed by strict dieting. But anorexics and bulimics also drift into bulimarexic behavior. The discovery that purging or vomiting makes it easier to indulge a disordered appetite becomes and irresistible but guilt-inducing temptation. The secrecy and self-hatred that result cause victims to withdraw from their friends and family. They become so addicted to the behavior that they opt out of social contacts so that they can binge and purge unobserved.

Bulimarexics may be distinguished from anorexics and bulimics by the emphasis they learn to place on the vomiting or purging. Eating gradually comes to serve principally as an introduction to the main event—the expulsion or expurgation.

> A 30-year-old executive described to us how she coped with the constant anxiety she felt about her daily round of business meetings. "I keep dozens of small packets of saltines in my desk, in my purse, and hidden all over the building. Right before I have to talk with someone, I stuff a few crackers down, slip into a bathroom and bring them up again. Somehow the routine helps me get through the day."

Our experience with patients indicates that the appetite disorder becomes symbolic of emotions that are felt but cannot be directly expressed. People who long to be loved but feel rejected may turn to food for comfort. They then punish and cleanse themselves by purging, a gesture that symbolizes both anger toward themselves and against the people who reject them.

There are other needs met in the binge-purge cycle, the most frequently reported being a brief sense of well-being that follows the episode. Many bulimarexics see their symptoms as an opportunity to totally let go all restraint, thus compensating themselves for their sense of being over-controlled in the rest of their lives.

> An anxious salesman told us how he relieves tension. "There are certain restaurants I have found that have bathrooms with an outer door I can lock. I go to these restaurants when I'm in the mood and really relax and enjoy the meal, knowing that I can get rid of the food fast, before I leave.

Unfortunately, the behavior itself quickly becomes addictive, and instead of gaining control, bulimarexics lose further control of their lives. This may set the stage for a variety of emotional disorders, especially chronic depression.

There is a special case of pathorexia that afflicts certain athletes and professionally beautiful people such as dancers and fashion models. These are people who have a great deal of their sense of identity, well-being, and security invested in their physical prowess or appearance.

Their success depends upon consistently winning in fierce competitions, and they have learned to be very disciplined with regard to training and diet in order to preserve their victor's edge. Sometimes athletes and dancers discover that they improve their performance by starving off fat and lean tissue while maintaining their strength through strict workouts of the muscles they use most.

The lost weight allows them to improve their speed and stamina or qualifies them to compete against lighter competitors. But the starving also triggers the appetite, as their bodies strive to regain lost substance. The change in appetite is unexpected and unwelcome. These intensely competitive people find themselves in another struggle, one that they have no preparation for. The result, frequently, is an attack of bulimia which usually changes to bulimarexia.

Athletes and dancers who seek help for their eating disorder feel that they are faced with an unpleasant choice between giving up an addiction or lowering their performance, and so, risking their careers. In our clinical experience, performance is too precious to be sacrificed, and pathorexia is accepted as the price of victory. The situation is similar for models. When they discover they can be more successful if they look more cadaverous, they accept semistarvation as the cost of staying in business.

It is a very human trait to choose visible, short-term gains over invisible long-term risks. For many people, a few years of forced vomiting seems trivial when compared to success in competition or prominence and fame as a celebrity.

It seems to us an awful irony that many men and women who are regarded as talented or beautiful and serve as role models to others live in a state of semistarvation and suffer the painful consequences of chronic malnutrition.

We do not know how long performers have endured pathorexia. The secrecy that has been the rule until recently may have casued generations of people to believe that they were alone in this behavior. Or perhaps our twentieth century culture has created stresses that lead many people to adopt extreme measures that only a tiny minority felt driven to in the past.

JEFF

Jeff became bulimarexic with the help of his softball coach. A good slugger, Jeff's liability was his slowness in running the bases. Each time Jeff was put-out, the team's coach would make a point of speculating on what the score might be if Jeff was "twenty pounds livelier."

Then Jeff came down with a serious stomach virus that lasted two weeks and left him ten pounds lighter. To everyone's surprise, Jeff was visibly faster in his first game back. Even his girlfriend complimented him on his sleeker appearance.

It was all Jeff needed. He lost, through dieting, another ten pounds and started running on days when there were no games. Jeff, who had never before given a thought to what he ate, was watching every bit. He found that the pizza and beer suppers that followed almost every game, and that had once seemed as much fun as the game itself, were now occasions of inner conflict—until he learned to throw up as soon as he got home.

When Jeff sought treatment a few months later, he was vomiting after each meal. He had become obsessed with his softball statistics, his figure, and his wardrobe. He had completely lost sight of his established identity as a carefree, husky hitter who left finesse and grooming to his less well-endowed friends.

Oral Expulsion Syndrome

This is one last form of appetite disorder that occurs occasionally. We believe that entertainer Glen Campbell was the first person to broadcast to the world the technique of losing weight by chewing food and spitting it out instead of swallowing it. We have found that a few people who experiment with this behavior are now addicted to it. They spend hours doing it in secret and, in time, develop intense anxieties about swallowing. As a consequence, they have become isolated, fearful, and seriously malnourished.

Not much is known about Oral Expulsion Syndrome. We do not know how common it is, who does it, or how many people who try it become addicted. We can see aspects of every other form of pathorexia represented in the behavior. We come to think of it as a low-key, low-profile pathorexia, the kind that a disciplined, cautious person might get caught up with. The following case study is a composite of some of the examples we have seen.

GLADYS

Gladys developed OES at age 37, shortly after her husband left her for a younger and, Gladys presumed, thinner woman. She began dieting furiously with a determination that was fueled by her anger at being abandoned. Soon, however, she developed an aversion to swallowing. "I went from having to force myself to swallow to believing that if I swallowed I would choke," she told us.

Because she was no longer consuming anything, Gladys felt free to put whatever she fancied in her mouth. Within a few weeks, she was spending all of her free time chewing or looking for food to chew. As her neurosis intensified, she began to fear that even the food juices she involuntarily swallowed were contaminating her.

Anorexia, bulimia, and bulimarexia are physically and psychologically debilitating disorders. The ill effects of starvation, bingeing, laxative abuse, and vomiting vary from person to person. Upsets in body chemistry, potassium deficiency, tooth decay, sore throat, liver damage, rectal bleeding, heart functioning, and chronic fatigue are common.

In 1983, the popular singer Karen Carpenter died from heart failure that was reportedly caused by a combination of starvation and laxative abuse. This happened at a time when she had regained a good deal of weight, and she was thought to be well on the road to recovery.

Most female victims experience some loss of menstrual function if there is significant weight loss. The inherent malnutrition slows tissue replacement. Cuts and sores heal more slowly. Forced vomiters sometimes develop infected abrasions on their hands from involuntary bites incurred while gagging themselves with their fingers.

Psychologically, the effects are seen in the gradual breakdown of honesty and sincerity. This begins with lying and deceit to conceal binges and stealing and shoplifting to finance them. The growing sense of worthlessness may trigger sexual adventurism. But the most common behavioral change is withdrawal from social contacts and increased involvement with the cycle of overeating, purging, fasting, or excessive exercise.

Gradually, even everyday activities such as shopping or being seen in public may become difficult. The disabilities may snowball until the severely pathorexic person lives in a world clouded with depression and imprisoned with anxiety. At last, the lonely victim seeks professional help or is forced into treatment by despairing parents or a judge.

Although there are many, many cases where these disastrous consequences have occurred, we should not lose sight of the fact that there are also people who have forms of pathorexia that, while they are potentially hazardous, do not appear to be especially handicapping. We have had brief consultations with many people who admit to a variety of appetite disorders but who claim that they feel fine. Some popular weight loss programs look to us like barely concealed forms of anorexia, bulimia, and bulimarexia.

We believe these people are living dangerously. We know they are closing their eyes to reality. But we know, too, that their personal experience with pathorexia has been more positive than negative.

Some eventually abandon the behavior after a few weeks or after many years. Others hear about the dangers from other people and then seek treatment. Karen Carpenter's death caused many people to get help they never before believed they needed. We hope this book will be the trigger for change.

Below, we have reprinted a questionnaire we use to screen patients. You can use it to rate yourself. Note that the scoring is not quite as straightforward as you might suppose. In many questions the answer *seldom* is rated as healthier than *never*. This is because everyone experiences some appetite upset, and denying oneself completely is less healthy than living with a normal weakness.

Appetite Disorders Questionnaire

Circle the answer that best describes you:

		Often	Sometimes	Seldom	Never
3	1. Do you have eating patterns that you suspect might be abnormal?	3	2	0	1
2	2. How frequently do you eat when you are not hungry? 2	3	2	0	1
3	3. Do you go for long periods without food when busy with other things? 2	3	2	0	1
2	4. Have you made unsuccessful attempts to lose weight by dieting? 3	3	2	0	1
3	5. Are you especially attracted to breads/sweets? 2	3	2	0	1
	6. Do you suspect that you are especially susceptible to the following aspects of food?				
3	smell 3	3	2	0	1
3	sight 3	3	2	0	1
2	thought of food 2	3	2	0	1
0	7. How frequently do you eat far more than your body needs before you feel full? 2	3	2	0	1
0	8. Do you feel uneasy if you cannot reach for a snack or drink between meals? 0	3	2	0	1

		Often	*Sometimes*	*Seldom*	*Never*
9.	Can you easily fall into long conversations about recipes, diets, restaurants, and other food-related topics?	3	2	0	1
10.	Do you feel tormented by your love/hate feelings about eating?	3	2	1	0
11.	Have you ever maintained an abnormally low weight through strictly disciplined eating because you were afraid you would lose control if you tried to eat normally?	3	2	1	0
12.	Do you avoid eating in public and then eat secretly, shortly afterwards?	3	2	0	1
13.	Can other people easily influence you to eat even when you are still digesting a good meal?	3	2	0	1
14.	Do you reach for food to tranquilize you and then feel remorseful after you have eaten?	3	2	0	1
15.	Have you secretly binged out of control in the past year?	3	2	0	1
16.	Have you followed a binge with:				
	induced vomiting or purging with laxatives or enemas?	6	4	3	0
	punitive fasting?	3	2	1	0
17.	Do you exercise to compensate for food you have eaten or plan to eat?	3	2	0	1

		Over 6	*3-5*	*1-2*	*0*
18.	How many close blood relations (siblings, parents, aunts, uncles, grandparents) have been diagnosed as alcoholic, diabetic, hypoglycemic or obese?	3	2	1	0

19

Scoring and Interpretation

0—20 points:	Healthy appetite
21—30 points:	Hazardous appetite
31—40 points:	Moderately disordered appetite
41—66 points:	Severely disordered appetite

Use this questionnaire to clarify appetite and eating problems. Notice that occasional indulgence is more *normal* than rigid compliance with healthy behavior. The scoring is based on clinical studies but is intended to be suggestive not definitive. This is not a diagnostic test.

3
overweight and obesity
what it really means
to be heavy

"From my point of view, being fat has always meant
having to say you're sorry."

This chapter provides an overview of obesity and includes definitions and descriptions of popularly accepted views of the obese state. We also discuss conditions that may play a role in the causes of obesity. We conclude with a review of the consequences of obesity.

Throughout history, the female body has been an object of admiration and desire; the subject of artists, poets and writers. Some of the great masters—Michelangelo's angels in the Sistine Chapel, Renoir's bathers, the nymphs of Greek mythology, and the Venus de Milo—portray women with robust, full figures.

These works of art show beauty that is sensual, sensitive, compelling, and timeless. Yet many Western women would not express satisfaction with the Venus de Milo's measurements of 37-26-38. Instead, they strive for the "perfect" 36-24-36 form or even the "delightful" 31-24-33 measurements of the model "Twiggy," who created a sensation in the 1960s with her unprecedented slenderness.

This quest for thinness, this desire to be light, is not universal, for obese women have also been highly sought after in many cultures at various periods of history. Some African tribes lock their pubescent females in fattening-huts where they are denied exercise and receive extra rations of food for as long as two years. This practice produces an overweight woman who symbolizes the well-to-do status of her family.

Other cultures and connoisseurs discriminate in their preference for the location of fat deposits. *Steatopygia* (large buttocks and heavy upper thighs), a well endowed bosom, or both with a small waist are classically fashionable choices for the female shape.

The pursuit of these proportions has led women to try a variety of devices and has made them submit to mutilations in order to alter their natural physique. Corsets and waist cinches caused fainting, rib fractures, and permanent distortions of the respiratory system, yet remained in vogue for generations and can be seen today in the costume of the Playboy Bunny. Around the turn of the century, some women had ribs removed in order to achieve this shape. More recently, silicone injections and breast implants have replaced the padded bra and bustle, revealing again an unceasing determination to conform to current ideals.

Thus we see that the admiration of the female figure, while universal, is subject to much aesthetic interpretation. What is praised at a given place at a given time will be sought after by those women who do not naturally possess this currently "perfect" shape.

Clinical interpretations of *obesity* are as varied as are cultural norms about what is attractive. Described below are some serious and not so serious methods for judging girth. Throughout this book, we repeatedly emphasize our concern that beliefs of what is overweight and obese must be determined individually, focusing on hereditary and health factors. The material that follows demonstrates the controversy that exists in defining obesity.

One common method of determining the relationship between ideal weight and height is this: 100 pounds for the first 5 feet plus 5 pounds for each additional inch. A similiar formula also states that if you subtract your waist measurement from your height and the result is less than 36 inches, you have a weight problem. A third equally as general a method says that one is overweight if, when lying on one's back on a hard, flat surface, the stomach prevents a ruler from being placed from the breast bone to the pelvis. At one time, television commercials told us that if we could "pinch an inch" it was time to buy a certain sponsor's cereal.

These methods seem naïve when held up to scientific scrutiny, and they have little relationship to beauty. We certainly know that some people are very healthy AND very attractive at a variety of weights. In one of the above methods, a slight curve in the spine would allow for a great deal of weight to be put on the hips before a state of overweight would show up. None of the aforementioned methods takes musculature or age into account, and they reflect only the crudest of aesthetic values. To use such simplistic formulae to determine proper weight is foolish and potentially hazardous.

Scientific attempts to specify criteria for obesity have been equally varied, but have typically focused on the percentage of body weight made up of fat deposits.

This has been done with instruments that measure skinfold thicknesses around the body—a grown up version of the pinch an inch technique—and by using mathematical formulae that include body weight in air, body weight in water, and body volume, determine the percentage of fat. There are also sophisticated electronic and surgical techniques that calculate very precisely the ratio of fat to lean tissue.

The Metropolitan Life Insurance Company published, in 1959, a chart of ideal weights that was the first one commonly used by health professionals. The tables offered a range of weights for various heights that people could interpret, based upon their own understanding of their body structure. It was widely but wrongly believed that these charts provided an accurate measure of how much a person should weigh for optimal health. In fact, the figures averaged about 15 percent below the mean-average weight of most healthy Americans, and the statistics were used to accuse millions of people of imprudent indulgence.

It wasn't until 1983 that new tables were published that contradicted the old charts and endorsed an upward expansion of the range for normal weight. While the new charts are improved, they are still based upon a population of insurance customers, they do not take into account age, and they are certainly not applicable to all individuals. We believe that they are still too vague and biased to be especially useful. Further question has also been raised as to the influence of smoking on weight and longevity.

Some of the most revealing statistics about the relationships between weight, age, and health have come from a study of over 5000 adults in the town of Framingham, Massachusetts, who have been given careful physical examinations every two years since 1950.

This immense enterprise has shown that only a minority of Americans conform to the Metropolitan Life "ideals" and that the mean weight for adult men and women of average height in Framingham is twenty percent higher than the tables' recommendations. The average man stands 5 ft 7 in. tall and weighs 168 lbs., and the average woman stands 5 ft 2.5 in. tall and weighs 142 lbs.

Nationally, Public Health Service statistics show that in recent years American men averaged 5 ft 9 in. in height and weighed 172 lbs., while women averaged 5 ft 3.6 in. tall and weighed 143 lbs. And we know from census data that these people, especially the women, are likely to live longer than any Americans before them.

In addition to discovering a great deal about the health and well-being of the population at large, the Framingham Study also correlated weight and mortality. The scientists discovered that even though heavier people have higher blood pressure and other medically hazardous conditions, they have to be much heavier than was popularly supposed to be a greater risk for an early death. Both men and women need to be at least 30 percent over the norms for their height to be considered a health risk by reason of weight alone.

Because we believe that it is nonsense to burden people with the label obese unless their health is potentially in danger, we use the 30 per cent cutoff as an initial measure of obesity. The following graphs show average weights for heights that were derived by combining data from a number of sources and shows our own rough guide to minimal obesity which is 30 per cent over those means.

It is important to recognize that the criterion for obesity used in these graphs is at best imprecise. We are using weight to indicate fatness, and that relationship is only approximate. Persons with substantial muscular development may be heavy without being obese, while others can be obese at lower weights.

We repeat that there are no simple measures of obesity. It is essential to assess each case individually to decide whether or not a person is a health risk because of being overweight.

Note, too, that the obese weight for men and women of the same height differs by as much as ten pounds. This is because the percentage of womens' body weight that should be fat is roughly double the amount for men. Although there is much variation and overlap in this statistic, it is reasonable to expect healthy women to be softer and rounder than men.

Today's fashions seek to deny this natural trait, and the figures in the table are vastly different from what is generally considered attractive. It is a

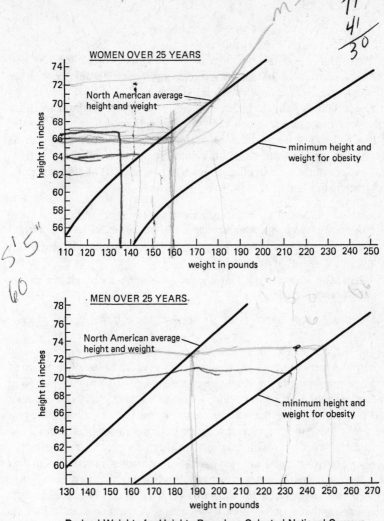

WOMEN OVER 25 YEARS

North American average height and weight

minimum height and weight for obesity

height in inches

weight in pounds

MEN OVER 25 YEARS

North American average height and weight

minimum height and weight for obesity

height in inches

weight in pounds

Derived Weights for Heights Based on Selected National Surveys

real and widespread tragedy that so many people are unable to accept their perfectly healthy bodies because they conform to biology and not to *Vogue* magazine.

Finally we need to consider one other factor that is generally ignored: the effect of age on weight. The Public Health Service and Framingham studies confirm the belief that as people become middle-aged, many of them gain weight. This is not a universal phenomenon, however, and therein lies the problem that causes so much pain. Thoughtless people, both lay and professional, argue that because some persons retain an adolescent shape throughtout their lives, everyone should stay thin. '

This simplistic attitude ignores the immense differences in personality and physique that bring so much variety to our culture.

In Chapter 8 we explain in some detail that the human body can be categorized according to three major characteristics that are inherited from parents and are not subject to change. Each of us is a blend of all three traits. The characteristics are:

1. A tendency to be soft and round and have substantial fat deposits. This is called *endomorphy*, and people who are high in this trait are called *endomorphs*.
2. A tendency to be heavily muscled. This is called *mesomorphy*, and people high in this trait are called *mesomorphs*.
3. A thin, bony, skeletal body. This is called *ectomorphy*, and people like this are called *ectomorphs*.

People who are about average on all three of these traits are called *midrangers*.

The effects of age vary with the type of body a person possesses. Endomorphs experience the most change, ectomorphs the least. The nature of this change is a slow gain in weight up to around age 35 in women and 50 in men, then a leveling-off period, followed by a slow losing period, beginning around 60 years of age. Because these changes affect the mean averages, young adults using the graphs can subtract 1.5 lbs for each year under 25 in order to get a closer approximation of their mean weights for their height.

Many environmental and psychological variables interfere with this process with changes in diet and activity levels being the most significant. Endomorphic people clearly tend towards obesity, especially in middle age. Acknowledging that special liability and acting to minimize health hazards rather than pursuing unrealistic aesthetic goals can make enormous differences in their sense of well-being.

The Causes of Obesity

"I know what causes obesity—it's everything I ever did or ever was!"

Established obesity is almost an irreversible condition, but our culture places such a high value upon slimness that millions of Americans spend their lives struggling fruitlessly to be thin.

Obesity is a complex phenomenon that has still not yielded itself to scientific investigation, though the literature is rich with research attempting to isolate the causes. With the exception of 5 percent of the cases which are attributable to physical dysfunction and hereditary diseases, there are no apparent causes for obesity, but research has revealed the significance of certain potentially key factors in understanding some obese populations. These factors are reviewed below.

As we will discuss in more detail in Chapter 4, a major discovery in the late 1960s, and then confirmed in the early 1970s, showed that fat cells are developed at certain critical periods of human growth. In infancy and adolescence and in pregnancy, the body's inherited potential for fat cell development is mobilized, and *adipose tissue* (a fancy name for fat) is made. The amount of this growth depends upon nutritional and environmental factors. These factors may cause the genetic potential to be unfulfilled or overdeveloped, according to individual circumstances. Fat cells also develop during pregnancy, and more may appear when existing ones grow to their maximum size. Whenever this occurs, it creates a permanent addition to the body's tissue. Fat cells can shrink, but they do not disappear.

Studies indicate that there is a relationship between multiple pregnancies and the development of adult-onset obesity, but the cause of such a phenomena is not immediately clear.

Perhaps fat is developed by pregnant women because of the presence of fat-promoting hormones in their bodies that are needed by the fetus. Or pregnancy itself could permanently alter the need for and use of food. It is also possible that nature tries to endow mothers with more fat so that they will be more resistant to infectious diseases and so better able to care for their children. Or enviromental changes may be responsible. Many women with small infants find it necessary to be in and around the home, exercise less, and spend more time closer to and tempted by food. Or self concept may be altered once one becomes a mother. If this change reflects an abandonment of lithe and sexy adolescence and the adoption of a more serious and stable figure that suits becoming a mother, then weight gain could well be influenced by the "motherhood self-image."

The physical and mental stress of being pregnant and dealing with postpartum depression may create the kind of arousal state that appears to accompany overeating. Finally, the work of caring for a new family member and the stress of adjusting to the change may also generate the need for extra stamina, which is achieved by storing extra fat.

Another cause of obesity is a hereditary predisposition to fat. A clear relationship has been demonstrated between genetic factors and the occurrence of obesity in animals. And it has been consistently observed that big parents have heavy children, even when the children are raised in foster homes. This leads most experts to assume that what is true for animals also holds true for humans. It seems fair to claim that genetic factors interact with social and environmental ones in the development of obesity.

Because we are all familiar with the natural human tendency to seek simple comforts like food when we are troubled, much research has been directed toward finding a link between emotional distress and obesity. Original studies conducted by scientists in the 1950s found a connection between anxiety and eating. It was therefore widely assumed that fat people ate because they were anxious. More recent work has failed to confirm consistent relationships between size, appetite, and emotions. Most contemporary investigators agree that obese people eat the same or less food than their thinner peers.

Some recent research has revived speculation that anxiety, depression, and stress are arousal states that are critical to the onset of obesity in some people. Reports from professional counselors and research scientists have described how people gain weight when they are upset and lose it again under stable life conditions. Some therapists see the use of food as a compensation for life's upsets, replacing what seems to be missing in life, and soothing, calming, and covering up daily stresses. But we know, too, that there are people who do just the reverse of this—they lose their appetites when they are troubled, sometimes becoming dangerously thin.

It has been our observation that people under stress have a tendency to do the opposite of what is good for them! Thin people stop eating, fat people go on binges. This is entirely consistent with the research on body types that we have discussed briefly above and will refer to in more detail in Chapter 8. Soft, round, endomorphs seek comfort in food and human contact. Bony ectomorphs lose their appetites and retreat into isolation.

Other studies have suggested that obese people, especially obese women, use fat as a shield to hide behind. That is, the fat makes a statement to the world about what they can and cannot do. It may protect them from certain social and cultural obligations, because few people expect a fat person to date or have an active sex life.

The fact that most obese people do, in fact, have normal sex lives, and marry and bear children, has barely dented the power of this widespread assumption. Many people still believe that being fat totally limits social opportunity. Heavy people are apt to be bombarded with unwelcome suggestions about how they could improve their fortunes.

> "My mother and grandmother are pretty heavy, but my dad is very thin. He keeps telling me I wouldn't have to worry about dieting if I'd just run 35 miles a week like he does!"

Finally, two promising areas of research on possible physical causes for obesity bear discussion. The first concerns studies of how the body generates heat from food, and the second investigates why metabolism is slowed down in certain obese persons.

It has long been speculated that mammals may control their weight by raising body temperature and burning off excess food in a process known as *thermogenesis*. Scientists recently confirmed that this indeed occurs and isolated the sources of thermogenesis in what are called brown fat deposits.

Brown fat, which is named for its color, is found in small deposits in rodents and other mammals, including humans, around the neck and chest. It has been most frequently associated with animals that hibernate and is known to play a role in survival at very low temperatures. Experimental data suggest that another function of brown fat is literally to burn off excess food so that it does not have to be stored in fat deposits. This may be accomplished by raising body temperature locally and radiating away unneeded energy.

This phenomena could account for the fact that many people never alter their adult weight regardless of how much they eat. Heavy people appear to have less brown fat than average weight people, and what they do have seems to work inefficiently. Studies are underway exploring techniques that could increase thermogenesis and permit obese people to burn off their excess fat. We look forward to further developments in this promising research.

The second fascinating new theory of obesity proposes that a deficiency of an enzyme with the strange name *ATPase* may predispose certain people to weight-gain by lowering their resting energy expenditure by as much as 25 percent. Obese people typically have 20 to 25 percent less ATPase than do people of normal weight. The more obese the person is, the lower their concentration of ATPase is likely to be.

A consequence of these lower levels of ATPase is to alter caloric efficiency in favor of obese people, who burn fewer calories than normal-weight people when they perform the same amount of activity.

The reason this happens seems to be related to an important metabolic process known as the *sodium pump*, which maintains different concentrations of sodium and potassium ions across certain cell walls throughout the body. It has been shown that obese people have lower pressure differentials across cell membranes than do normal weight subjects. This means that the sodium pump consumes less energy in obese people, who therefore survive on fewer calories.

These findings lend further credence to the claim of many overweight persons that they do *not* eat more than other, slimmer, members of their families—a claim that has found consistent support in public health studies conducted around the world over the past 20 years, studies that have contradicted our conventional wisdom, and for that reason have often been ignored. Now, however, the evidence is too conclusive to ignore, and we can state that many obese people eat less than the nonobese, and periodic dieting or fasting often has the long-term effect of making heavy people heavier.

In the light of these developments, it seems we should revise our whole focus of attention. Given the fact that almost everyone in Western societies eats more than is needed to survive, we should, instead of looking for why some people are fat, search for the mechanisms that keep most people thin. As scientists discover that heredity, fat-cell deposits, hormone variations, thermogenesis, and other metabolic effects contribute to obesity, it becomes clearer that will power and morality are irrelevant in determining how much fat a person is destined to carry.

The Consequences of Obesity

"I am so tired of being judged first for my weight
and second for my personality."

There are numerous consequences related to being overweight, all of them negative. In most cases, the more overweight one is, the more serious the consequences are. One generally inescapable handicap of obesity is prejudice.

Surveys show that even fat people agree that being heavy is evidence of poor character. It is easy to see how that translates into self-critical attitudes.

Furthermore, some of the strongest social prejudices against fat people are held by health professionals who know how hard it is to change obesity. Surveys of physicians indicate that many of them view heavy people as lazy, self-indulgent, and indifferent about their appearance, weak-willed, emotionally disturbed, or "jolly slobs" (slob defined as dirty, dumb, and lazy). Verbal harrassment of the obese is a frequently reported public occurrence. Even children are victimized.

Heavy children are less likely to be among the most popular in school where athletics are often a social focus. Among young people, being pretty or muscular are very strong norms. Lack of ability to conform to these values may lead to ostracism and cause lasting emotional scars. Later, the obese person may find it particularly humiliating to be the one friend in a group of old friends who is not, for example, asked to be a member of a wedding party, who discovers that he or she is welcome only when the whole group gathers and is the last to find a partner when the gang grows up and pairs off.

ANNE

At five-foot two-inches and 196 pounds, there was no question that Anne was a soft, round person! And a lively and attractive one too. But Anne was everyone's friend and nobody's lover. Men often sought her counsel and cried on her shoulder, but they never dated her. When she came to us for help she was thirty and a virgin—a combination that depressed her and saddened us.

We offered support, warned her away from crash diets, and urged her to be patient. As a trouble shared is a trouble halved, Anne felt better and regained some of her familiar spontaneity. She also joined a bowling league, where she was able to demonstrate convincingly that her shape did not impair her athletic ability. Six months later, when next we heard from her, we learned that she had improved her score both on and off the alley. She had a boyfriend she was delighted with, and she assured us repeatedly that he was well worth waiting for.

Anne's parents, who were also heavy, were fond of reminding her that they, too, had had a long search before they met. Judging by the snapshot she showed us of her boyfriend, if the relationship proves successful, Anne's own children will very likely face the same task of seeking acceptance as fat people.

Overweight seems to carry more serious social consequences for women. The following statement was made by Dr. Helen De Rosis at a seminar in Washington, D.C. entitled, "Overweight: Its Special Implications for Women":

> A man, even if he weighs two hundred fifty to three hundred pounds, does not incur the public adverse regard that a woman does. Men are supposed to be big. But women are not.

In recent years, heavy women have begun to recognize that the unfair discrimination they experience can be overcome. Fat consciousness-raising groups have formed at many women's centers, and a glossy fashion magazine, *Big Beautiful Women* (see Bibliography), has built up a 300,000 copy circulation.

It is our impression that the status of fat people may parallel in many ways that of Black people in 1950. We welcome and endorse every move to acknowledge their needs for respect and fair treatment.

Nevertheless, it is still important to recognize that the physiological disadvantages of obesity, while they in no way warrant discriminatory attitudes, may be serious and, in some cases, life threatening.

For many years, excess weight has taken a comparatively greater physical toll on men than on women, as it adds to their already existing greater risk of heart disease and stroke.

Obesity has been associated with some twenty-six medical conditions that may account for as much as twenty percent of the mortality rate. It is related to increased incidence of hypertension, gall bladder disease, stroke, heart disease, and diabetes.

For people at risk, weight control has been proposed as the most viable method for correcting disease states and prolonging life. It is for this reason that obesity cannot be looked at merely as a social handicap or a matter of aesthetic preference.

Because of the higher incidence of obesity in women, it is important to look further at the health complications unique to them. Women not only suffer from the general consequences. They are also subject to a variety of reproductive system difficulties: decreased fertility, increased likelihood of spontaneous abortions, prolonged and difficult childbirth, and general menstrual problems. Higher rates of uterine cancer have also been reported in obese women. And breast cancer now appears to be related to obesity—certainly it makes detection more difficult.

There are also statistical correlations between diabetes and weight. We are not sure whether diabetes causes weight gain, or weight gain causes diabetes, but studies suggest that a *moderate* overweight state increases the likelihood of diabetes and a severe overweight condition raises this risk thirty times. We know, too, that prudent weight loss can reverse these trends. Gallstones and gallbladder disease are also much more common among overweight women.

Finally as heavy people age, their weight may aggravate joint problems and create spinal problems, especially among women. There is also evidence that women who are obese fall more easily and are more likely to be hurt when they do fall.

4
who's at risk?
the chance for fat

---

*"I wanted someone to see what I was doing
and say, 'STOP!' But no one noticed, so on I went."*

We now turn to a review of the populations that have a higher risk for developmenting obesity and pathorexia.

Recent research has yielded some important concepts that must be considered if obesity and eating disorders are to be prevented. To begin with, we can better understand the problem by examining two separate groups: those with adult-onset obesity and those with juvenile-onset obesity.

The juvenile-onset obese are defined as people who have become at least 20 percent above the average weight during infancy or adolescence. This is not an easy statistic to discover, because childrens' heights and weights are even more variable than they are for adults. But most of us believe we know what we mean when we describe a child as fat. There appear to be three main factors leading to juvenile obesity. The first contributing factor is heredity— the child of one obese parent has a 40 percent chance of becoming obese while the risk increases to 80 percent if both parents are obese.

The second factor that appears to contribute substantially to juvenile-onset obesity is early overnutrition. Fat babies may be called cute, and mothers may receive compliments with respect to how "healthy" their babies look, but a rotund baby is far from a picture of good health. In actuality, the weight put on during infancy is likely to predispose that individual to a lifetime of being overweight.

The third contributor to early weight gain relates to emotions. When we pacify babies with bottles and young children with sweets, they soon learn to display this type of behavior on their own. If a baby cries or a child takes a fall and we respond by comforting the child with something sweet, it should not surprise us to find this same child coming home from an upsetting day at school and cleaning out the refrigerator. Stress and anxiety continue to rank among the most plausible contributors to weight gain in both juvenile- and adult-onset obese groups.

We will examine the causes of obesity in two separate groups based upon age of onset, because juvenile obesity influences individuals' physiology for the rest of their lives.

Although obesity is a widely researched area, until the 1970s, few investigators focused on age of onset as a critical issue for their studies. This is due, in part, to the relatively recent discovery of the relationship of juvenile-onset obesity and the production of fat cells. A critical time for the development of fat cells occurs between birth and age 2. A second period begins in early adolescence. The amount of fat cells produced during these periods is related to heredity, nutrition, and activity level.

Early-onset (juvenile) obesity is thus associated with an increase in cell numbers. Adult-onset obesity, in most cases, however, represents simply an enlargement of already existing cells. Once one has become an adult, new fat cells are developed only in response to a massive overfeeding for a prolonged period of time. The juvenile-onset obese individual who reduces weight will continue to have more adispose cells than those who have never been overweight and more than those who have become heavy, for the first time, as adults.

Decreases in the body fat of juvenile-onset obese individuals are accompanied by reduction of cell size without changes in cell number. An international authority on obesity, Dr. Judith Rodin, writes:

> Thus, even in children, once a particular adipose cell number is achieved, it cannot be decreased by dietary restriction, and these (one time fat) children usually become overweight adults.

The significance of the number of fat cells must be understood. It appears that fat makes fat. The larger and more numerous one's adipose cells, the greater becomes the ability of the body to produce and store more fat. This means that *people who are substantially overweight have a greater risk of further weight gain than do normal-weight individuals.* The more cells one carries, the greater the physiological predisposition to fat. And, remember that the number of cells cannot be diminished.

When examining the etiology of adult-onset obesity, the first suspect is always juvenile-onset obesity. Was this person actually obese as an infant or child and is simply returning to an enlarged state as programmed by his or her fat deposits? If the individual is truly overweight for the first time, we then look for other causes.

One factor that appears to contribute significantly to obesity is conscious-appetite restraint or, rather, the removal of such restraint. Many people are constantly, actively, and consciously resisting food. Under certain circumstances, their motivation to resist is reduced—marriage, pregnancy, and depression are frequently cited examples—and control of eating is essentially lost. Thus, a woman who has been a normal weight all of her life may become obese during pregnancy, not only because the pregnancy changes her metabolism, but also because the knowledge that her figure will soon become enlarged no matter what she eats gives her permission to abandon all restraint in eating.

Stress, anxiety, and depression have repeatedly been assumed to have a direct relationship to adult-onset obesity. However, our own research has found that the only emotional handicap linked fairly consistently with obesity is depression. and even that is by no means a universal connection.

Finally, there are also complex interrelationships between obesity and one's socioeconomic status, race, and ethnic origins. About one-third of all lower-class adults have been identified as obese, compared to only one in twenty upper-class women and less than a fifth of upper-class men. According to scientists who study populations, lower-class black women are at the greatest risk of all. Roughly 50 percent of them have skinfold measurements above the 85th percentile for women in general.

We suspect that poverty, cultural values, and cultural change all have an impact on weight. Poor immigrants (including poor blacks moving to northern cities) exposed to relatively inexpensive, high-caloric food may increase their intake, and in doing so induce obesity in those of them who are physically at risk. Cultural values in these populations may not include prejudice against being overweight or obesity—indeed a soft roundness in a woman and heaviness in a man may be viewed quite positively.

Also, cultural change may result in the loss of healthful, traditional dietary customs that are replaced by the seductive messages of advertisements for processed food. The impact of all these factors diminishes with assimilation and education.

The table below summarizes the risks for obesity and includes factors discussed both within this chapter and elsewhere in the book.

HIGH RISK OF OBESITY—Juvenile-onset

1. Being female
2. Parent(s)/Grandparents obese
3. Overfeeding in infancy
4. Excessive use of food to cope with stress or as a reward for achievement

HIGH RISK OF OBESITY—Adult-onset

1. History of juvenile obesity
2. Being female
3. Parent(s)/Grandparents obese
4. Long term depression and or stress
5. Long term history of restrained eating
6. Massive overeating for a sustained period of time
7. Lower socioeconomic status
8. First or second generation American or subject of major cultural change

The brief questionnaire following summarizes and weighs the severity of certain risk factors for obesity. The interpretation that follows provides a general sense of whether a tendency to become obese exists.

Ideally, those who score over 16 points but who are not now obese should take all precautions necessary in order to prevent obesity from developing.

Rate Your Risk of Obesity

Give yourself:

1. 5 points for each obese parent or -10 if neither were obese _____ pts.
2. 5 points if you are a moderate social drinker _____ pts.
3. 15 points if you were fat as an infant or adolescent, -15 if you have never been heavy _____ pts.
4. 5 points if you frequently turn to food when upset _____ pts.
6. 5 points if you frequently feel depressed _____ pts.
7. 5 points if life has recently been unusually stressful _____ pts.
8. 5 points if your life revolves around restraining your appetite (constant dieting) _____ pts.
9. -10 points if you exercise four or more times in a week _____ pts.

Scoring and Interpretation

-35 – 0 points:	It is highly unlikely that you will develop fat
0 – 15 points:	A minor chance that you will have a weight problem
16 – 25 points:	A modest tendency toward becoming overweight
26 – 40 points:	You are a considerable risk for becoming overweight
41 – 55 points:	You are in the high risk group

Anorexia, Bulimia, Bulimarexia

"I couldn't leave the house for any reason,
without giving myself an enema first!"

Pathorexia—severely disordered appetite—is most frequently a disease of childhood and adolescence primarily affecting females. The conforming, undemanding, and unassuming child is often the victim. These children seem as though they cannot do enough to please their parents and are typically attractive and good students—too good for their own good.

Pathorexic children are good because they feel insecure. A common reason for developing the disorder is a conscious or unconscious effort to keep a disintegrating family together. Pathorexia creates a problem that parents can work on together, thus stalling the family discord that the children fear so much.

DIANE

Diane's anorexia began imperceptibly—shortly after her parents started to talk about divorce. Never anything but thin, Diane had still not entered puberty at fourteen. Even she did not realize that she was skipping meals and spending hours staring into space.

Finally, when she had dropped to 56 pounds, a teacher called her parents to draw attention to their daughter's condition. Her mother and father recognized the fact that Diane was starving herself to death and hospitalized her.

Diane's depression that had caused the loss of appetite gave way to anorexia during the hospitalization. She was a difficult, disruptive patient at first, but began to eat after two months of family counseling. Her parents always came and left the counseling sessions together, and they increasingly supported each other's attitudes and opinions.

Only in retrospect did Diane and her family recognize that her crisis had been the beginning of the parent's reconciliation.

Sometimes children may feel compelled to behave in an overly conformist fashion because they sense that one or both of their parents need them to be well-behaved to maintain the parents' shaky convictions about the right way to live.

When this happens, the child becomes a parental figure. This can easily create a stress overload in an already insecure youngster. The good child also frequently reports not knowing how to cope with the give and take of peer relationships. The child can only respond to others by playing strictly by the rules.

Many pathorexics are unable to express anger effectively, especially toward a parent or an authority figure. In most households, adolescence is associated with a difficult shift of authority from parents to maturing children. In pathorexic families, there is little overt evidence of conflict, anger, or a desire for new experiences. Instead, the child's disordered appetite becomes a metaphor for other appetites: fear of and desire for sexual expression, fear of and desire for closeness in relationships with others (especially parents), or a fear of and desire to simply let go of all emotions, be they joyful, angry, or just loud! Often, the family has the outward appearance of being the epitome of middle-class normality.

"My mother is such a great lady, I can't believe I'm telling you I hate her now. But when I think of all the ways she made my life so perfect, so soft, so cushie, I get furious. Now I can't handle anything by myself. I don't even know who I am!"

Sometimes, however, it is the complete absence of middle-class norms that causes a child to become the family caretaker.

> Gretchen's parents divorced when she was an infant. Her mother, a talented musician, helped make ends meet by singing in nightclubs and bars. Unfortunately, her career was handicapped by her tendency to get drunk. Gretchen's childhood was terrorized by the men her mother brought home, some of whom made sexual advances towards Gretchen as she approached puberty.
>
> Gretchen resolved that she would grow up to be everything her mother was not. She was a model child at home—cleaning, cooking, and maintaining her room spotlessly. She was an excellent student, and worked hard to become a good pianist. But she could not overcome her fear and disgust of men and of physical contact of any kind.
>
> Gretchen became bulimic after she got a job at a doughnut shop. Her fellow workers were very social, held parties often, and dated among themselves. Gretchen could not bring herself to join in the fun. Instead, she took home boxes of day-old doughnuts and binged alone in her room. The more isolated she felt, the more she turned to food for comfort—starving herself for three or four days after each binge to avoid weight-gain.

Examination of the family life of pathorexics often reveals intelligent and capable mothers who gave up their career aspirations in order to be excellent parents. This struggle for excellence may be measured by the proper development of their children. In order to experience success, these well-intended mothers become enmeshed in all aspects of their daughters' lives.

Fathers, on the other hand, are typically immersed in their own careers and remain emotionally distant. Nevertheless, fathers' values, while rarely expressed, have a powerful impact on their families. For example, if a child overhears the father commenting on the mother's expanding waistline, the remark, though lightly intended, may register as an imperative to stay slim, in the teenager's mind.

Two dynamics with negative consequences may thus be set in motion for the teenage child. First, the child must be thin to avoid Dad's disapproval. But in remaining thin, there is direct competition with the mother, a state that neither parent nor child is likely to miss.

While Dad's comments may have been intended as helpful or were benign, they generate both fear and hostility in children, and they do nothing positive for mother's ego! The children may feel more isolated and more conflicted about their roles as young adults and about their status within the family. Always chronic pleasers, the children are in a no-win situation.

> "I know if I didn't get good grades, my folks wouldn't say anything but they sure are happy with my straight A's. I hope I never disappoint them."

The about-to-be pathorexic children feel that their activities are controlled, while their emotions are ignored. Their secret life with food is both a metaphor of, an escape from, and a rebellion against the barrenness of their lives. They compensate by bingeing, purging, and starving until they are discovered or allow themselves to be caught. (Some bulimics "forget" to flush the vomitus in their parent's bathroom bowl.)

The discovery of a pathorexic child may have a convulsive effect on the family, especially when it results in hospitalization of the child. We have likened it to a delayed action bomb, ticking away for months or years until it explodes and exposes the family to a danger that has been present, but ignored, for so long.

As well as the need to be good and only function by the rules, pathorexic children want self-perfection. The children's obsession with thinness and their fear of fat is part of a determination to maintain a perfect record of control, proving to themselves that they can manage everything they feel responsible for. Through "constructive starvation," they sublimate both their fear of failure and their anger of a world that demands so much of them while giving them little in return.

The profile of the pathorexic child includes:

High Risk for Pathorexia

1. Being female.
2. Being undemanding even from infancy.
3. Consistently achieving excellent grades.
4. Never talking back to parents.
5. Limited emotional expression, especially of anger.
6. Becoming obsessed with appearance/perfection.
7. Living in a home where there is much marital discord or living with the fear of losing a parent through illness.
8. Experiencing a severe setback in personal or interpersonal goals.
9. And finally, becoming ritualistic and obsessive about food.

Rate Your Child's Risk of Pathorexia

Give your child:

10 1. 10 points if female, -10 if male.   *10* pts.

5 2. 5 points if he or she has always been undemanding and cooperative.   _____ pts.

10 3. 5 points if he or she is generally a perfectionist, adding another 5 points if his or her appearance must always be perfect, and adding another 5 if his or her school grades must always be perfect. Subtract 5 if your child is willing to "let some things go," and subtract another 5 for less than perfect appearance or grades.   *5* pts.

5 4. 5 points if he or she expresses little or no anger.   _____ pts.

5. 10 points if either you or your spouse have been ill, missing from home, or incapacitated for a prolonged period of time.   *0* pts.

6. 10 points if you and your spouse are currently having, or have recently experienced, marital problems.   *10* pts.

10 7. 10 points if he or she has recently experienced a traumatic event such as a move away from friends and school or if he or she has been abused or sexually harassed. Give 20 points if both have occurred.   *20* _____ pts.

10 8. 10 points if there is a history of obesity in the family; -10 if there is no history of such.   *-10* pts.

10 9. 10 points if he or she often struggles to lose weight.   _____ pts.

10. 5 points each if either you or your spouse are preoccupied with 1. food, or 2. physical appearance. (This could total 20 if both parents are preoccupied with food and appearance.)   *20* _____ pts.

5 11. 5 points if he or she frequently speaks of hating his or her body.   *5* pts.

Scoring and Interpretation

30

-35 – 0 points:	Pathorexia highly unlikely
0 – 25 points:	Little likelihood of pathorexia
26 – 56 points:	Moderate risk ⟶
57 – 87 points:	High risk
88 – 115 points:	Expect to see danger signs

Danger Signs—Pathorexia in Progress

1. Binge eating, no eating, and/or secretive eating.
2. Withdrawal from friends and all social activities.
3. Obvious change in eating patterns.
4. Constant preoccupation with food—cooking and shopping for others.
5. Frequent, frenzied, and excessive exercise.
6. Evidence of forced vomiting, frequent use of laxatives, diuretics, or enemas.
7. Rapid change in weight, especially weight loss.

5
avoiding trouble
prevention is better
than cure

"If only I hadn't started bingeing and purging.
I feel like an addict. Even when I'm eating normally
and not vomiting, I feel like it's lurking right over
my shoulder waiting to snare me again."

Both obesity and pathorexia are resistant to cure once they have taken a firm hold upon the individual. They are emotionally and physically hazardous diseases, and some of the known treatments carry substantial risks with only limited results. This chapter presents a case for the prevention of obesity and pathorexia and makes some suggestions on how to accomplish those goals.

Appetite disorders are a serious concern to literally millions of Americans. Severe obesity is linked with hypertension, cardiovascular disease, increased risk of cancer, aggravation of degenerative joint diseases, and economic and social handicaps. There is overwhelming evidence that once one has become obese, one will remain so. Those who do reduce, fight a continuous battle with food and often return to the obese state.

"Every time I sit down to a meal, something inside me makes me feel
like this is my last chance to be full, so I tell myself, Go eat all you can."

The act of dieting itself appears to be an emotionally difficult endeavor.

Depression, irritability, anxiety, and hostility are reported much more frequently in dieters than in non-dieters, regardless of whether they are obese or of normal weight.

Cure after cure has failed the obese person, with weight loss nearly always being followed by substantial weight increase. Even radical surgical interventions that shorten the intestine or reduce the size of the stomach cannot make good a lasting guarantee of slimness. In addition, the risk of complications—such as diarrhea, malnutrition, liver disease, bacterial overgrowth, kidney failure, arthritis, and choking—make such measures far from utopian.

The pathorexic faces at least equivalent risks. Death through self-imposed starvation is certainly the supreme loss, with the risk of heart failure from potassium imbalance an ever present possibility. Further risks include all the physical symptoms related to malnutrition, including kidney disease, menstrual problems, metabolic changes, and mood swings. Additional complications that are a direct result of purging behaviors include stomach ruptures, the inability to defecate without external stimulation, sore throats, tooth decay, scarred hands from pressure exerted during forced vomiting, diseased and swollen salivary glands, and burst blood vessels around the eyes.

The depression, irritability, and anxiety found in obese populations while they diet becomes a way of life for pathorexics. Their distorted body image may keep them in a constant state of near panic. Their lives are lived for food. Their days are planned around food—either how to get it or how to avoid it. It is a true, full-time obsession.

Statistics on "cure" rates are not readily available for pathorexia. The National Association of Anorexia Nervosa and Associated Disorders (known as ANAD) estimates that only 50 percent of all recovered pathorexics will remain free of symptoms, 25 percent will live with reduced behavior problems, and 25 percent will not experience any meaningful remission following therapy. These figures agree with our own results and thus point to a severe and lasting problem that we would rather prevent than treat. It may be helpful to think of the recuperating pathorexic the way we think of the non-drinking alcoholic—in a state of recovery but always vulnerable, unable to ignore the potential for a return to the substance abuse, either food or drink.

The prognosis for the obese to remain permanently "normal weight" is bleak. The hope for a totally "normal" life for the pathorexic is guarded. It is clear, then, that the best case for prevention lies in the failure of available restorative therapies—a topic we will examine in more detail in Chapters 6 and 7.

> "I started by only vomiting up the junk foods and letting three meals a day digest—then I thought, wouldn't it be great to lose weight faster? God! if I had only known before I began what a mess I was getting into. . ."

The first step toward prevention identifies the populations at greatest risk. Parents, educators, therapists, dietitians, and other professionals can then work together to short-circuit the mechanisms that promote these pernicious disorders.

While large gaps remain in our understanding of why obesity and pathorexia develop, we do know enough to design profiles of high risk groups. If these problems are a result of how we live and what we expect from ourselves and our children, controlling them may lie in altering our lifestyles and expectations before we are stricken.

At the same time, it is important not to ignore the low-risk population. Increasing numbers of men are becoming trapped in pathorexic addiction. Middle age, "normal weight" men who are anxious to regain or maintain their youthful silhouettes are developing anorexia, bulimia, and bulimarexia as they fight the battle of the bulge.

There is much evidence that our society's values with respect to weight and shape have become more rigid and critical in the last two decades. Although a variety of body shapes have been fashionable in the past and women have felt it vital to their well-being to conform to fashion, only recently have the majority of Americans felt the crushing passion to live by the norms of *haute couture*.

Barbara "Babe" Paley, the socialite wife of the President of Columbia Broadcast System coined the phrase "You can never be too rich or too thin." The slogan caught on, despite the well publicized fate of the billionaire Howard Hughes, who died alone in a state of extreme emaciation.

A century ago Mrs. Paley's influence would have extended no further than the tiny minority of leisured rich. Today, her slogan is the watchword of tens of millions of Americans. The media constantly reinforces it by insisting that virtually everyone portrayed in movies and on TV appear ectomorphic regardless of the content of the film or program, creating the impression that only thin people are normal and only thin people can be successful.

On the other hand, we live in an economy that has a huge stake in selling us things we don't really need—including food. The food-industry profits depend on marketing processed food so tasty and attractively packaged and advertised that we will add it to our diet.

The conflict between the pressure to eat and the pressure to be thin has been heightened in recent years by the shift in our perception of the ideal American woman from images of apple pie and motherhood to a Supermom, capable of handling both career and family responsibilities. This expansion of womens' roles has clearly aided women by enlarging their opportunities, but it has also increased the stresses upon them.

Women are expected to be disciplined, authoritative, and in some cases, "masculine," when they are at work, but they are expected to remain feminine and yielding in sexual and social settings.

The thin woman is thought to be best equipped for this dual role. Her straight body, with minimally developed curves, wears the executive three-piece suit most successfully. For social occasions, she can switch to frilly fashions that exemplify the decorative side of her identity. Missing here is the acceptance of the full, soft, adult female form that many women are genetically ordained to inherit.

In order for preventive measures to be effective, powerful social and economic forces will have to change, with a primary focus on children's nutrition education. Teachers in all the grades and educators of future teachers and health professionals must pay attention to principles of sound nutrition and healthy exercise. Parents, teachers, and therapists must avoid food-centered reward systems for dealing with stress or disappointment. ("If you will stop crying you can have a lollipop.") Sweets or junk food should not be rewards for good behavior either.

Health maintenance issues must be marketed for children in a way that competes successfully with the glamorous images that are projected for junk food and exercise-free entertainment. Health professionals need to develop models that teach good nutrition in new ways, ways that increase compliance among consumers. Families aware of the risks of overnutrition, underexercise, and overachievement are well set to cope with the legacy of twentieth-century affluence.

Preventive Strategies

Unfortunately, a number of the risk factors for appetite disorders and obesity cannot reasonably be altered. With regard to obesity, if one is or has a female child with a familial history of being overweight, certain precautions are recommended. Special care should be taken to be sure that infants are neither overfed nor underfed. Overfeeding produces additional fat cells that the individual will never be able to get rid of and that will always be ready to store unneeded, surplus fat. Underfeeding may produce a pathorexic response that will result with the starving child being unable to control appetite and being constantly obsessed with food.

> Maria, an obese, 30-year-old patient, always knew that she had begun her constant search for snacks and sweets at about age three. But she had no idea why. At Thanksgiving, conversation at the family get-together turned to reminiscences about early childhood events. Maria's mother told how she had put Maria to bed with a glass bottle each night, until, at age two-and-a-half, the bottle was broken in a mishap that soaked the mattress and left jagged glass in the bedding. The nightly bottle in bed ceased abruptly. The anecdote was a watershed in Maria's life. From that time on, she had a reason to resist overeating that crystallized her desire to be grown up and in charge of her life. She lost weight steadily and permanently.

When infants cry or children scrape their knees, parental attention and physical affection are the healthy ways to soothe them. While a bottle may be the quickest, most effective way to induce quiet in an infant and a cookie restores peace in the house, as long-term strategies, they are likely to induce a dependence on food. Parents of high-risk children would do well to avoid these feeding responses.

Positive substitutes for food are the healthiest training we can give our children. When they are very little, the best intervention is cheerful smiles and hugs for the sad or frightened child. As they get older, parents can involve them in activities that distract them from the unpleasant conditions. Avoiding the use of food for such coping is an important first step toward the prevention of overweight children; using physical activity as a preferred outlet is a further step toward good health.

Obese parents face a double bind. Not only are their children in a high-risk group, but they themselves might wish to change their established behavior patterns that may have contributed to their own obesity in order to avoid negative modeling for their children. We acknowledge with respect the courage and determination it takes for a heavy mother to involve her children in health promoting athletic activities and dietary habits when she was never encouraged to do so herself.

Those who are at high-risk for adult-onset obesity are well advised to take precautions toward maintaining a state of good health. Women with either family or personal histories of obesity should not assume that during pregnancy they can "eat for two" without a risk of unwanted weight gain. Special attention needs to be paid to maintaining a healthy pregnancy weight, both for the fetus and the mother. Too little weight gain robs both of them of necessary nutrition and may actually cause deformities in the fetus and lower the potential intelligence of the child. With too much weight gain, the mother may have a more difficult pregnancy, delivery, and future with weight control. Toxemia is also a frequent problem when too much weight has been gained. Keep in mind that pregnancy is a time when fat cells can emerge and become permanent additional tissue.

Those people whose weight is maintained through continued restraint, or a lifetime pattern of avoiding certain foods, know that an extended break from that restraint is likely to lead to obesity.

It seems that restrained eaters become trapped in a dilemma in which there are no pleasant alternatives. They must always hold back or become fat. It may be that restrained eaters are actually fighting their natural or hereditary physiques. We discuss the importance of accepting hereditary characteristics as a preventive measure for pathorexia as well as for obesity throughout this book. For perpetual dieters, we offer the suggestion that *relaxed restraint*, which minimizes total prohibitions but always monitors intake of appetite provoking treats, may allow them to maintain better long term control.

When depressed and when under stressful circumstances, women in high-risk groups appear likely to gain unwanted weight. Awareness of these dangerous times helps make it easier to fend off overeating behaviors. For high-risk people who are experiencing a great deal of stress, it may be wise to seal the refrigerator or take other precautions that will remind them that right now food is hazardous to their health!

Prepare to cope with stress in ways that do not involve eating. Seek counseling, take assertiveness training, run, swim, even shop for clothes. These are established techniques that work well, both alone and in combinations.

> "I guess I was just stupid. One time I forgot to flush the toilet and my mother saw the, you know, vomit. After that, she asked me a whole lot of questions, and finally I had to tell her the truth."

The pathorexic child is harder to identify in terms of predicting risk. As we mentioned earlier, this is most often a problem for girls. Parents who have a "perfect" daughter who never confronts them or disappoints them often find it difficult to question her about her health or their role as parents. Her record of exemplary behavior protects her like a shield from any implication that problems may exist. However, this tendency toward goodness may be the first clue offered that beneath the surface there is turmoil.

> An adolescent anorexic who was trying to survive on a regimen of lettuce and ketchup told us, ''When I was in 2nd grade we had to sit with our hands together. I used to imagine myself being perfectly still, not moving a muscle, and getting hundreds on all my tests. I still think about that when I'm tempted to skip on my diet.''

Permitting a child to be less than perfect is healthy. It is fine to have goals and dreams for children, but it is not fine to push those ideals on a child who does not fight back. It is not a good idea to decide what a child should become and then set out to control the child's life in order to see that narrow dream come true.

> Mrs. Reed's first three children had always seemed destined for success. Sure enough, two became doctors, like their father and uncle, and the third became an architect. Her youngest daughter, Mary, never had her brother's or sister's energy or drive, and Mrs. Reed decided that Mary would never leave home or marry. Mary would always be with her.
>
> She subtly discouraged Mary's obvious talent for math and science while constantly reinforcing her artistic ability and rewarding her domestic skills.
>
> When we met Mary at age 25, she had lived two lives for eight years. Outwardly demure, restrained, and conforming, she sincerely believed that her mother needed her to help look after her now sickly father. She had never learned to drive and was a prisoner in her own home.
>
> Mary's second life was lived in her bedroom. There, she submerged her consciousness in a never changing world of science fiction novels and bulimarexic behavior. She used garbage bags to sneak vast quantities of food into her room and reused them to sneak the vomitus out, dumping them in the trash barrels of an apartment building next door. When she was not eating or reading, Mary made delicate, hand-crafted greeting cards, which she gave away or sold, and grotesque illustrations of maimed monsters, which she kept for a while and then destroyed.
>
> We suspect that Mary's mother knew more about her daughter than she ever admitted. But both of them had become victims of the mother's desire to have Mary stay home. Mary had failed to develop the social

skills necessary to survive in the outside world, and the mother wa
dependent on Mary's presence that she sabotaged every move her o\
children made to help their sister grow up.

There are three parental curses that are often innocently inflicted on children:
the admonition, "Just do your best!"; the wish, "All we want is for you to be
happy,"; and the slogan, "If a thing's worth doing it's worth doing well."

Each of these familiar bits of homespun wisdom can easily be inter-
preted by a susceptible young person as minimal expectations for daily life,
rather than goals to be aimed for. When this happens, children come to
believe that they must feel happy, work themselves to exhaustion, and do
everything perfectly the first time. This combination induces severe stress and
an almost certain sense of personal failure. Teaching a child to expect life to
be a mixture of successes and disappointments is excellent preventive medicine for a gamut of disorders, not the least of which is pathorexia.

One or both parents of pathorexics are often preoccupied with physical
appearances. Their children frequently feel that they can and should continually strive to look attractive. All too often, they develop ideals based upon
photographs in fashion magazines that are totally unattainable outside of a
studio. As a consequence they begin to form erroneous ideas about their looks
often thinking of themselves as fat or deformed if they cannot fit into ultra-
small clothing.   TRIGGER

Parental remarks about the appearance of the pre-teenager, whether
positive or negative, may not be in the child's best emotional interest. Simply
telling a perfectionistic girl that she should "knock off a few pounds" can set
up a pathorexic response. As Susan Wooley, an expert with an international
reputation in this field said on the Donahue TV show, "This is the first
generation of Americans to be raised by Weight Watchers mothers."

> "When I'm on a diet, I think about food all the time. I wake up thinking
> about breakfast. When that is done, I think about lunch for three straight
> hours, and on, and on. I wish I could think about sex once in a while, like
> other people my age!"

We have repeatedly observed that some diets actually cause eating disorders,
and we discuss this in more detail in the next chapter. Diets that produce a
starving organism increase the body's craving for food and cause people to
lose their ability to detect appetite. Fashion magazines and dieting literature
continuously market thinness to teenagers. Parents who want ideal children

Society

also give them the message, both verbally and nonverbally, that they are expected to be thin. If thin is in and stout is out, what do you do with a naturally rounding body? Why starve it, of course!

Naturally plump children who have inherited their shapes, may go to great lengths to distort their own bodies in order to comply with society's current norms. Self starvation and purging behaviors that begin as dieting techniques set up a lifetime of obesity problems or pathorexia.

The message here is to accept ourselves as less than perfect and to be realistic about our own and our children's physical appearance, not attempting to change what nature has given us. Prevention rests on giving permission to find and experience healthy outlets for all appetites, for food, for love, for independence, for security, for expression, for solitude, and for caring and being cared for.

This does not contradict what we stated concerning the prevention of the onset of obesity by taking appropriate precautions for high-risk groups. Simply stated, one should strive less for the stick-thin figure of a fashion model and substitute, instead, a healthful lifestyle. This means good nutrition, adequate exercise, and plenty of reinforcement of the notion that one's well-being comes from the pursuit of happiness and not from being a doll-like person, appreciated only for one's appearance.

6
marketing thin
the merchants of narcissus

"The diet clinic helped me to lose weight. Now I'm neurotic about
fat and scared to death of food."

The fight for thinness, a battle that consumes millions of people, has created
armies of professional and commercial services that offer a wide range of
advice to the fat- and weight-conscious. The slogan "You can never be too
rich or too thin" takes on a different meaning when we review the world of
weight control. You need to be rich indeed not to risk impoverishment by
purchasing many of the services aimed at making you too thin!

The quest for a fashionable figure has seemed, until very recently, to be
a reasonable goal if reasonably pursued. This has created a huge marketplace
in which all kinds of interested parties vie to sell services. They range from
dedicated scientists, concerned health and mental health professionals, and
ethical drug suppliers and food manufacturers, to out-and-out charlatans who
trade on the naïvety and despair of their customers.

In the long run, few of these supporting forces, whether honorable or
not, are offering true value for money. It is quite possible that a person would
be better off spending $15.00 for a mail-order, plastic running suit to sweat

in, than to spend $1,500.00 for inpatient treatment at a prestigious teaching hospital. It all depends upon what the buyer does with the merchandise.

By and large, weight loss is a self-limiting activity. Even though "over-weight" people are virtually unanimous in claiming that they would be happier if they were lighter, the effort required to reduce and stay reduced increases with time, while the added benefits of being thinner decrease as more weight is lost.

What usually happens, long before the ideal weight is achieved, is that the value of losing another pound is perceived as less painful than the cost of necessary deprivation. At this point, no more weight will be lost, the future will look bleak and punitive, and refeeding will soon begin, with a return to the original weight, or to a heavier weight, as the end result.

Weight reduction schemes offer the public a relatively restricted group of options. They are marketed in an endless variety of packages, constantly recreating the impression that something new and different has become available. The underlying techniques used include the following: drugs (prescribed and over the counter), surgery (intestinal, cosmetic, and oral), diets, behavior modification, psychotherapy, group support, exercise programs, and gimmicks. Let us take a look at each of these in turn.

Drugs

The pharmaceutical treatment of obesity is by far the most appealing route to thinness, as it boasts of an effortless weight loss. Also, the association with medicine implies that a cure is being accomplished.

Most of the potent drugs in use are available only by prescription. Weight obsessed patients have long been a stable source of income for physicians in general practice, but they are a goldmine for doctors in a less respected branch of medicine, bariatrics, who have made weight loss their speciality. These practitioners use three major categories of drugs: amphetamines and their derivatives, thyroid hormones, and exotics—preparations of various kinds of drugs with negligible or non-existent medical value but with exciting sounding potential.

There is no question that the amphetamines do promote modest temporary weight loss. There is equally no question that the continued use of these medications fails to produce further losses. Termination of the treatment is followed by weight gain, and maintaining the use of these drugs is dangerous.

They are marketed under a variety of proprietary names *Dexamyl, Fastin, Pondimin, Preludin, Sanorex,* and *Tenuate* are popular preparations. All of them are closely related, chemically.

Despite years of research on animals and people, the action of these medications is still not fully understood, but their use initially reduces appetite and may increase energy expenditure.

Because they induce conditions in the body that mimic a state of alarm or arousal, they may inhibit the digestive functions, causing the body to use fat rather than food for energy.

It is possible that some of the anorexic effect of these drugs is a consequence of their inhibition of the salivary glands, which creates a dry mouth, makes food less palatable, and results in a loss of appetite.

Both of these mechanisms have only temporary effects. The body soon draws on its immense recuperative powers, learns to adapt to the chemical, and restores digestion, salivation, and appetite back to normal, thus preventing any more loss of tissue.

It is possible their effect is short lived because appetite reduction is a side effect rather than a principal action. They may work by resetting the body's preferred weight, or *set-point*, to a slightly lower level. Once the new weight is achieved, appetite is restored to normal. If this is how they work, further weight loss can only be achieved by increasing the dosage. This raises the hazard of an ever greater dependence on chemicals.

There is one amphetamine that is available without a prescription and that is apparently just as effective as those that are not. It is called *phenylpropanolamine*, or *PPA* and is more familiar to most consumers as the decongestant in such cold remedies as *Contac, Robitussin CF*, and *Vicks Formula 44D*. It is also approved for sale as an appetite suppressant and is the "active" ingredient in a host of preparations like *Dietac* and *Dexatrim*. These are sold over-the-counter in pharmacies and supermarkets. *PPA* is often misleadingly advertised by mail-order companies as a sure cure for fat. Typically the ads will say "Approved by the Federal Government," implying that this represents a guarantee of effectiveness, when in fact it means that the substance *may* work, but is unlikely to be harmful if used as directed.

If it has been your own experience that decongestants have significantly reduced your appetite, you want only to lose a few pounds, and your blood pressure is normal, PPA may be all that you need. If any one of these prerequisites is missing, amphetamines are not for you.

If you do use PPA, make sure you don't take a double dose by treating a cold and your appetite at the same time!

There are two other substances which are sold over-the-counter as appetite supressants: bulking agents and topical pain killers. The former— *Metamucil* and *Pretts Tablets* are popular ones—are taken before meals and swell up in the stomach, creating a sense of fullness that is supposed to inhibit excess eating. The pain killers use *benzocaine* to reduce sensation in the mouth and make eating a less rewarding activity. We believe that benzocaine is more usefully employed to ease the pain of sunburn and the sting and itching of insect bites. As a weight reducing device, you can find it in *Ayds* candy.

It is our experience that none of these substances provides a lasting change in eating patterns or weight. It seems that their principal function is to enrich the people who manufacture and sell them. Two other nonprescription medications are also used for weight loss: laxatives and diuretics. But these are not openly sold for that purpose. Instead, they are adopted by desperate people to compensate for overeating. Unfortunately these substances often work where others fail, creating dependency upon drugs that cause severe and lasting physical damage when they are used inappropriately. Bowels may not move again without their stimulation.

Thyroid hormone, which occurs naturally in all healthy people, is another prescription medication that is still aggressively marketed as a weight reduction agent, even to people whose thyroid glands are in good working order. This practice is dangerous, as continued use may have the effect of supressing the body's normal secretion of this endocrine.

Thyroid medication is supposed to raise the metabolic rate and cause more calories to be consumed. In certain cases where a glandular problem exists, this does occur. For healthy people who are naturally heavy, the drug is of no value. The long and fruitless use of the hormone for weight loss by healthy subjects is a striking testimony to the willingness of patients and physicians to substitute wishful thinking for good judgment in the treatment of obesity.

Two current fads are *HCG* and *starch blockers*. These substances offer a lot based on limited research and have proved ineffective in the long run.

HCG is a hormone extracted from the urine of pregnant women, and is typically administered in a daily series of shots that are accompanied by encouragement to stay on a starvation diet! The rationale for this treatment is that weight change during pregnancy is apt to be long-lasting, therefore, if we mimic pregnancy and induce weight loss, a permanent change may be accomplished. Unfortunately, follow up studies have not demonstrated that HCG patients stay thin any longer than their peers in other programs.

Starch blockers make a virtue out of the familiar problems associated with eating beans! By concentrating into a medication the protein in certain beans that inhibits starch digestion, they prevent complete metabolism of carbohydrate. This causes malnutrition and possible weight loss accompanied by flatulence and an upset gastric system.

For people who derive much pleasure from eating, starch blockers may allow them to eat more without gaining weight. Overfed people may reduce to their normal weight without lowering their food intake. But for the majority of the would-be-thinner people, these pills are yet another technique to create semistarvation and its inevitable consequences, which we have repeatedly described already. As we write, starch blockers are off the market pending Food and Drug Administration approval.

Surgery

Surgical intervention for the purpose of weight loss is performed in three forms: cosmetic, gastric, and oral. The former seems to go directly to the heart of the matter—unwanted adipose tissue is simply cut out of the body. Unfortunately the procedure is less simple than it might seem.

Fat deposits are not isolated surplus tissue but a part of the living organism, joined to and embedded in and around muscles, nerves, veins, and arteries. It is possible, at considerable expense and some risk, to reduce the size of these deposits in the arms, thighs, and abdomen with skillful surgery.

Plastic surgery to repair disfigurement and to improve physical proportions has brought relief and renewed self-esteem to many people. But it is not yet possible to remodel a body so that the plain becomes marvelous, and any results may be only temporary. Fat slowly accumulates to replace the lost tissue, but the scars from the incisions are permanent!

Gastric intervention (stomach and intestinal surgery) is limited to grossly obese patients. It attempts to reduce digestive efficiency by shortening the small intestine or by reducing the effective size of the stomach. This should create a state of semi-starvation and corresponding weight loss. Both techniques have had mixed reactions—some truly grateful, newly thin persons, and some disappointed people who expected a lot and received a little, and a few fatalities.

It is not yet possible to predict who will benefit from this surgery. Despite careful screening of candidates, there are instances where patients have eliminated the possibility of weight loss following treatment by added consumption of high caloric food. Whether this represents a psychological or physiological response is not clear, but it is a remarkable commentary on an organism's investment in a certain size and shape. Over time, the small intestine may accommodate to its loss and once again digest as effectively as it did prior to surgery.

Recently, a research study that compared the emotional health of obese people who opted for and against surgery found that both groups were physically identical. However, the people refusing surgery were living full lives and were emotionally normal; those seeking surgery were emotionally less well, and lived restricted lives. The researchers concluded that the people who are most likely to seek surgical intervention are least likely to profit from it.

Similar commentary applies to a third physical intervention—jaw wiring. In this dental procedure, the patient's jaws are loosely connected with stainless steel wires so that biting and chewing become difficult or impossible. Other oral functions, like talking, drinking, and vomiting, are less seriously impaired. The semi-liquid diet that must be consumed is unlikely to have the calories that will maintain weight, so losses are incurred, again through a form of semi-starvation.

Many desperate people have found jaw wiring to be a route to a more acceptable physique. They endure the suffering (not to mention the humiliation) of an imprisoned mouth to enjoy the (temporary) satisfaction of a thinner figure. The professional literature lacks reports of long-term follow ups of this technique, but there is no reason to suppose it to be superior to other methods.

Diets

Because there is such a deep conviction in our culture that unusual fatness is linked to overindulgence in food, it is natural to believe that changing consumption is the most honest and righteous way to achieve weight loss. It is a short step from there to conclude that if people cannot control their intake alone, they need help from people who are better informed about what is wise to eat.

While there is merit in this assumption, there is also a fatal flaw. It lies in the failure to distinguish between guidance and control. We can all profit from education and advice, but we are much less able to profit from the regulation of a behavior as intimate and personal as eating.

Many people who have come to believe that their appetites are unhealthy seek to surrender their free will to an authority who will deliver them from themselves. But very few of us are so lacking in self-assertion that we seldom will follow an outsider's rules for long periods of time. So diets, from the scientific to the outrageous, are rarely followed for more than a short time. And the more rigid their requirements, the less amount of time they are followed.

A tiny minority of people who attempt dieting put themselves under the complete care of the medical profession and spend weeks, sometimes months, in hospitals or health resorts as patients. Here, they may be treated with carefully formulated and individually adjusted diets that incorporate the most up-to-date information available. Often, these diets will be designed to minimize the loss of muscle and other non-fat tissue, and for that reason are referred to as *protein sparing modified fasts* or *PSMF*.

There is some evidence that PSMF can fool the body into shedding more fat than muscle, especially when the diet is supplemented with a rigorous exercise schedule designed to maintain musculature. However such diets are hazardous if they are attempted without close medical supervision. This is presently an area of intensive study. There are indications that carefully balanced, high-quality protein diets may have important clinical applications.

Two popular, commercial, dietary aids should be mentioned: 1) food substitutes sold to increase non-nutritive bulk, and 2) liquid formulas designed to be complete replacements for normal meals. In the first category, research has shown that people quickly adjust to disguised changes in the caloric density or richness of experimental foods, so the body is not fooled for long by these substances. However, the psychological effect of tasty, low-calorie meals may be a little longer lasting and may help people maintain a regimen of semi-starvation. These meals will not, of course, create a sense of well-being in an underweight person.

The fluid-replacement diets share the same fate as all the other rigid modifications in eating behaviors: people, in general, abandon them after a few weeks and a few pounds are lost and gradually return to old eating patterns.

Non-food substances that mimic the taste and cooking qualities of sugar and fat have met with some success. If any prove to be delicious, inexpensive, and medically safe, they are likely to be viewed as a boon to food lovers and find extensive use. While it is hard to predict their effect, we may discover that candy and desserts with low calories permit some heavy eaters to indulge without unhealthy weight gain—perhaps getting a satisfaction similar to chewing gum.

Regardless of what may show up in the future, diets will always have an enduring place among reducing techniques, and they will owe it all to the fact that virtually all of the them work—for a while.

There are two principal reasons why short-term weight loss can almost be guaranteed: all diets lower the caloric intake so that some starvation occurs, and most of them impose a nutritional shock to the system that takes the body a couple of weeks to adjust to. Thus, both low-carbohydrate and high-carbohydrate diets will cause brief weight loss. If a diet is in any way diuretic, the loss of water will increase the effect of the nutritional trauma.

So we have the familiar experience of a brief success followed by disheartening failure. Because most people will attribute the success to the diet and the failure to themselves, the net effect is to reduce the dieter's already low self-esteem while leaving the diet and its author's reputation unblemished.

Year after year, the weight loss gurus recycle their familiar themes, and the womens' magazines publish varieties of quick weight-loss programs in issue after issue. Yet nobody points out that if even a fraction of these techniques really worked, we would be rightly described as the slim society. There would scarcely be a fat person left in the land!

It is clear that diets as alternatives to free will do not work, but some guidance is needed if we are to make healthy food choices. Dietitians are the helping professionals who are trained for this purpose. In a society in which, as we noted in Chapter 3 and devote more space to in Chapter 8, a major part of the economy is fueled by the sale of manufactured food of low nutritional quality, only the dietitians, working through the media, the schools, and the medical profession, keep us aware of the importance of the four food groups, the hazards of high fat consumption, and the dangers of overprocessed foodstuffs.

The collective voices of professional dietitians serve as a quiet but insistent counterforce to the barrage of expensive advertising that urges us endlessly to buy, to splurge, to indulge, to enjoy, and to risk our health for the benefit of the food industry.

In raising questions about the value of diets as methods for permanent weight change, it is important that we distinguish between diets that cause caloric deficiency and diets that end caloric overload. The former are fraudulent in proposing that a single diet, no matter how carefully prepared, can provide for the well-being of persons of varying age, size, health, and metabolic state. The universal warning "check with your doctor before you begin this program" is an escape clause that protects the authors from legal responsibility.

Ending overindulgence, on the other hand, is a much more difficult proposition. While there can be no doubt that many people abuse food, it does not follow that everyone with a big appetite or massive fat deposits is sick or abnormal. If the person's weight has not changed significantly in several years, and the blood pressure and the blood-sugar are within healthy limits, chances are that the individual is *defending,* to use a technical term, his or her proper adult weight.

As we discussed in Chapter 2, substantial "overweightness" does not necessarily decrease life expectancy, and big people are not necessarily over-eaters. Some people who crave food and eat a lot may be underweight individuals whose bodies are working to restore lost tissue, even though they are heavier than they would consciously wish to be. Or they could be compensating for depression, having found that carbohydrates temporarily relieve their chronic sense of sadness.

Although many individual differences are normal, and to be respected and not modified, problems arise when we consider the plight of people who have overeaten and become obese despite their bodies' genetic and regulatory mechanisms. Our clinical practice has included many clients who spent years substituting available food for absent affection. Latch-key children are an example, as they habitually fill the lonely hours after school with junk food, candy, and television. Others who experience family tragedies—death, illness, and ugly divorces, for example—often use the pantry as a surrogate parent.

There are also many people who are so nutritionally illiterate that they allow their choice of menus to be guided by advertising, convenience, and flavor—virtually without regard to content.

These people have grown fat and stay fat. They have a high risk for hypertension and diabetes, and present medical wisdom concludes that they would be better off thinner. Certainly they would be better off eating nutritionally balanced meals. Careful guidance, both dietary and emotional, is indicated here. Effective treatment must be long-term and individualized. No possible good can come of simple recommendations "to go on a diet and lose some weight."

Exercise

Increased energy expenditure as the route to weight loss has gained an extraordinary number of enthusiasts in the past decade. There is much evidence that this is a key factor in promoting health and preventing weight gain for many people. Physical fitness through physical activity is widely endorsed, representative of our cultural ideals, and is a logical corrective action for self-indulgent behavior.

How better to atone for years of indulgence than by hours of exertion! It may seem foolish, even anti-American, to propose exceptions to this concept, but we have come to recognize that the exercise fad is, in part, just another stick to beat the obese with. The fact is that not everyone can, will, or should find salvation in a sweat suit.

First, however, let us review the benefits. The human frame is roughly divided equally by weight between the limbs and the torso. The twentieth century has seen a steadily diminishing need for strong limbs. Enough muscle to get us from our cars to our kitchens and a reserve to take us upstairs to our beds could suffice for our needs. Technology has rendered our limbs almost redundant, faster than biology has been able to compensate.

Our response has been to shift from a nation of workers to one of exercisers. Through sports and active recreation, we find the mechanisms to remain healthy in an environment that tolerates sloth.

Exercise also helps reverse the effects of poor diet. Obese people with slow metabolisms and overeaters with disordered appetites can all experience an easier relationship to food if they maintain suitable activity. Aerobic exercise (and it is important to stress the need that it be aerobic, i.e. fat-fueled) increases the metabolic rate, reduces appetite, firms muscles, improves cardiac and respiratory function, burns fat, and keeps us out of the kitchen.

Just a few weeks of daily workouts of thirty minutes or so brings about these abundant benefits. The resulting sense of well-being is often quite intoxicating. Enthusiastic beginners resolve that they will never be fat or sluggish again; they feel that life has new meaning and value and that their pursuit of happiness has at last been successful.

While it is true that the mass discovery of the benefits of physical fitness has virtually guaranteed that our public health statistics are going to improve in the coming years, not everyone is able to enjoy these benefits. Many people who experience all the positive rewards of exercise still fall back to a familiar sedentary routine and regain the weight they have lost.

We believe that there are two major reasons for this: the first is based on population statistics, and the second on variations in body type.

North Americans and Europeans in the second half of the twentieth century are, at all times, influenced by the enormous rise in the birth rate that followed World War II. As this bulge of humanity moves from the cradle to the grave, it dominates, and will continue to dominate, our economic and social environment. What happened in the 1970s, and is continuing to influence the 1980s, is that babies born in the 1940s and 1950s have aged to the point where bountiful health is no longer an unearned benefit. As they pass their mid-20s, the strength, speed, and svelteness that graced their youth diminishes. Their response is typical of the work ethic that is still the keystone of our culture. They begin an endless struggle to hold back the march of time.

Today, we are still at the point where most people believe that earnest exercise is the price of well-being. And for many, it indeed is. Others of us, however, have accepted social and professional responsibilities that quite simply diminish the possibility of vigorous exercise. Torn between the multiple demands upon us, we relegate active recreation to a minor role. Regardless of the benefits it promises, there is a limit to how far we are willing to follow fashion.

The second major reason why not everyone will exercise is that only persons with certain kinds of physique find voluntary activity invigorating. As we describe in more detail in Chapter 8, the human body can be categorized according to three criteria: soft and rounded (endomorphic), square and muscular (mesomorphic), and thin and bony (ectomorphic).

The degree to which people take naturally to exercise depends a lot on how muscularly endowed, or mesomorphic, they are. Predominantly endormorphic and ectomorphic people are reluctant athletes, poor performers, and early quitters. The mesomorphs, on the other hand, cannot be kept home for long—their need to be active is constant, pressing, and dominant.

The search for slimness rarely takes these variables into account. While the inactive ectomorph is rarely condemned, the unmuscled endomorph, who finds no pleasure or success in competition, is continually urged to "get out there and exercise."

Of course, relatively few people have extreme forms of body type. Most of us are *mid-rangers,* with a blend of all three characteristics, but even so, our temperament is likely to reflect our most prominent body type. The amount of satisfaction we take in activity will be related to our degree of mesomorphy.

It is most unfair to regard everyone as a potential athlete. Sometimes the programs inflicted on the obese border on punishment. A recent "experiment" at the University of Pennsylvania seemed especially so. Heavy women subjects were required to pedal exercise machines while submerged to their necks in cold water. This humiliating regimen was continued for an hour a day, five days a week, for six weeks. No weight loss was recorded—probably because the poor victims' bodies avoided freezing by maintaining their fat stores.

This is a good place to note how cruelly our present culture treats endomorphy. Fat people suffer in three ways. High levels of refined carbohydrates, sugar, and fat in the typical western diet makes them heavier. Mechanization has limited their enforced daily energy expenditure. And fashion has identified them as homely. It takes courage to be "overweight" in America today, a courage that millions have sought by joining groups formed to aid in weight loss.

Group Treatment

Group treatment for weight reduction ranges from informal get-togethers among friends and neighbors to multimillion dollar organizations like Weight Watchers. They are formed by heavy people seeking support in the battle with their bulges, researchers collecting information, health professionals offering help, profit oriented corporations marketing programs and promises, and various combinations of all of them.

Some of the self-help groups have become international organizations. *Take Off Pounds Sensibly*, or *TOPS*, and *Overeaters Anonymous*, *OA*, have grown steadily for over twenty years and have been havens of help for many. *Weight Watchers*, the giant of the commercial operations, now operates all over the world. Other successful programs are tied to institutions and have gained in prestige rather than size over the years—the *Duke University* clinic is a good example.

Most of these operations have two things in common: they bring "overweight" people together, and they promote standard procedures to combat fat. An exception should be made with Overeaters Anonymous. OA is concerned with overeating not being overweight, though weight loss is not discouraged.

Our concern with these programs is that they are ready to offer service to anyone willing to join. The clientele is self-selected, and the assumption tends to be that if a person *feels* overweight then he or she *is* overweight, and treatment will be initiated. It follows that goals are established that are more often guided by cosmetics than by physiology, and the hazards of excess weight loss are virtually ignored.

The consequence of such procedures is that the programs may cause pathorexia in people who, prior to treatment, had no appetite disorder and were not clinically obese or unhealthy. The net effect of such weight loss is likely to be an aroused appetite, unwanted weight gain, panic, and a second round of treatment.

Irresponsible weight reduction procedures from which this sequence of events follows have a built-in bonus for the commercial operations. Customers frequently seek to be recycled through the program, unaware that the prior treatment they received contributed to their present misery. No weight loss program ever admits this. Most, in fact, stress the permanence of their results. But there is little, if any, evidence to back up their claims. They always welcome back old clients who want to start over.

We do not know how much the big operators depend upon repeat business. But to the extent that their programs create future clients by training people to unbalance their metabolisms, they are profiting by making people sick.

By and large, the group programs offer some mix of diet, exercise, and behavior modification, presented in a social context that blends mutual support with competition. Leaders who can inspire just the right mix of these ingredients create a highly motivating atmosphere in which dispirited fat people find acceptance, challenge, and renewed self-esteem.

Powerful, positive experiences, both emotional and physical are realized, and participants often learn to feel good about themselves. Some for the first time in years. Many success stories begin, "It started when I joined the _____ weight control program. . . ." Group treatments that maximize these gains and make careful assessments of individual needs may be excellent therapeutic mechanisms. There is a great need for caution in selecting programs, however, as many offer far more than they deliver. **Look very carefully** at the professional credentials of the owners and operators. In recent years, many programs have been set up by totally untrained people. Others have collected large fees from prospective customers and have then gone out of business overnight.

Behavior Modification

Behavioral treatments attempt to train people to abandon unhealthy eating behaviors and adopt healthy ones. The changes are accomplished by introducing a system of rewards, and sometimes punishments, plus alterations in the patient's environment. People are usually weaned away from junk foods and snacks, trained to eat reasonable meals at accepted mealtimes, and taught to develop activities that are substitutes for eating.

Many effective programs were developed using these concepts (we include one we call STEM in Chapter 10), and for a while it seemed that the key to the control of obesity would be found in the perfection of this approach. Long-term follow ups, however, were rarely done, and those that have been done, proved disappointing. Like all the other interventions, behavior modification was a short-term success and a long-term failure for most of the people who tried it.

We believe that the reasons for this failure boil down to two main issues. First, attempting to alter a healthy if possibly unfashionable organism mobilizes powerful recuperative responses that will restore the preexisting equilibrium. The body will demand weight gain. Second, most behavioral therapists have access only to the relatively superficial aspects of their patients' lives. When treatment ends, entrenched patterns of behavior reestablish themselves.

Behavioral treatments work best when early gains open the way to further improvements in living—for example, when successful sex therapy leads to an enhanced marriage. Losing weight might seem to fit this model very nicely, but for many people it does not. The early pleasure associated with being thinner usually gives way to a realization that life has not changed all that much, and staying thin turns out to be a constant struggle. Given this outcome, relapse is almost inevitable.

Only people who truly change their lives for the better, succeed in maintaining substantial weight loss but only for as long as their newly discovered satisfactions depend upon their staying thin. We are reminded again of how many women we have met who lost weight, met their husbands, married at the lightest weight of their adult lives, and then returned to their previous size.

Psychotherapy and Hypnotherapy

Mental health therapists are frequently sought out by overweight and obese patients on the assumption that an emotional problem has caused them to be fat. For people who have gained weight as adults and as a consequence of identifiable stresses, such a referral is entirely appropriate. It may also be wise to seek a psychological evaluation if only to rule out the possibility that adiposity is psychological and reversible.

Unfortunately, not many therapists are well-informed about these matters, and we have detected a tendency in the profession to presume that emotional health correlates with a fashionable appearance.

Therapists who can identify realistic physical and dietary goals and can then assist their clients over the emotional hurdles impeding them may be crucial figures in restoring or enhancing the patient's health. In the "buyer beware" climate that pervades psychotherapy today, finding a therapist who is both adequately trained and personally compatible is apt to be a matter of trial and error. We urge people who are seeking treatment to feel free to check a number of potential therapists and to ask direct questions about their knowledge of eating and appetite disorders before committing themselves to a course of treatment.

These cautions need to be reiterated more forcefully when applied to hypnotherapy—a healing art with a justified reputation for quackery as well as a core of qualified and effective practitioners. Treatment to promote weight loss is a stock-in-trade of virtually all hypotherapists, and short-term changes in eating behaviors are not difficult to achieve by using post-hypnotic suggestion. The effect is rarely lasting unless it is accompanied by therapy that brings insight, understanding, and emotional growth. These gains are unlikely to occur unless the therapeutic relationship is based upon more than a facility for trance induction. Check very carefully before seeking help of this nature.

Gimmicks

Last, and by all means least, we should mention, and quickly dismiss, all gadgets, gimmicks, and garments that are sold—almost always by mail-order—to "melt" fat in minutes a day without pain or effort. The utterly ineffective varieties on the market include items like inflatable pants, rubber corsets, and plastic overalls. Faintly less fraudulent, but no more likely to be effective, are the exercise wheels, rope and pulley devices, elastic cords, and cheap pedalling machines that are billed as being capable of transforming one's body, if used briefly but conscientiously on a daily basis.

While exercise does have a value in health maintenance, the mechanisms themselves have no special therapeutic effect. They are usually so cheaply made that they break before any benefit accrues from their use.

In this context we should mention two other kinds of mechanical exercisers—those that work and those that do not.

The first are the quality built stationary bicycles, rowing machines, and treadmills that are found in any well-equipped gymnasium and that may be purchased for home use. Such machines are costly but effective, and using them properly—which means with considerable effort—will improve physical fitness, and may induce weight loss. (Note: We do not include weight training equipment in this category because it is most often used for non-aerobic exercise which has no value for weight reduction.)

The expensive machines that do not provide meaningful assistance are the passive "exercisers" and massagers. Commercial slimming salons—establishments that are often no more than large-scale gimmicks—use these electric-powered rollers, vibrating belts, and whirlpools. While they are fun to play with, may give an invigorating massage, and even have value in physical therapy, they will not promote weight loss.

Similarly ineffective devices are saunas, hot tubs, mud packs, body wrappings, and all the other constantly changing offerings that wax and wane in popularity over the years. Enjoy them by all means, but do not imagine that they have benefit beyond the immediate sense of well-being and relaxation they create.

7
therapy for pathorexia
the search for understanding

"The first two therapists I went to couldn't believe
that eating was my problem. They wanted to talk
about everything else in my life except food!"

The appetite disorders that cause a severe underweight state or bizarre eating behaviors have not yet given rise to commercially oriented therapies. These disorders are still alien and a little scary, and their victims lack the visibility and familiarity that characterize the obese. As a consequence, when treatment is sought, mental health professionals are the most likely to be called.

This has served to preserve a cloak of secrecy and a sense of mystery over behaviors that in reality are neither uncommon nor as frightening as, say, chronic drunkenness or reckless driving.

The low level of public and professional understanding of appetite disorders leads to abnormal anxiety. Many therapists, aware that anorexia nervosa is a potentially lethal condition, are reluctant to offer treatment to a self-starving person. In contrast, they do not hesitate to accept a depressed patient who is actively contemplating suicide. Again, until recently, bulimia was believed to be a rare and dangerous phenomenon that was unlikely to be encountered in clinical practice. As a consequence, these expectations become self-fulfilling.

In the past, most pathorexics did not seek treatment, and those who did tended to be in extreme distress. Neither the professionals nor the public realized that behind facades of middle-class normality hundreds of thousands of Americans were existing in various states of semi-starvation or were engaging in massive overeating and purging cycles. And for the most part, the people involved in these practices thought they were alone, trapped in behavior patterns they could not change, and convinced that no one would accept them if they told the truth about themselves.

A major change in public awareness of eating disorders occurred in 1981 when many newspaper articles and television programs about bulimarexia appeared. *Newsweek*, in its year-end issue, facetiously referred to 1981 as "the year of the binge-purge syndrome." In some adolescent circles, girls who were known to vomit gained status, and the expletive *Barf!* became popular and gained a positive as well as a negative connotation.

Attitudes toward food and eating shifted dramatically with the growing awareness of how potentially hazardous eating disorders could be. Bingeing found a place in the repertoire of teenage activities that cause parents sleepless nights. It is too soon to determine what effects these changes will have beyond the fact that they have greatly increased the number of people who have contracted pathorexia.

A long time exception to the general ignorance of eating disorders has been the growing group of people who find relief in the care and understanding of Overeaters Anonymous, an organization modeled on the teaching and practices of Alcoholics Anonymous. OA members acknowledge the fact that when they are alone, they are powerless in the face of their desire to eat compulsively. They recognize that weight is not the issue: eating is the problem.

The parallels between compulsive eating and alcohol abuse are many and close, and the two organizations have helped many thousands of people regain lost self-respect and a sense of control over their lives. Most OA members are fat, but not all. There is much empathy, understanding, and support for all appetite-disordered people. OA has become a major therapeutic resource for pathorexics of all kinds.

It is important to recognize that it is a non-professional self-help group run by and for its members, who are all self-diagnosed compulsive eaters. They do not presume to make medical or technical judgments about each other. This fact represents both its strength and its weakness: strength, because all leadership is based upon personal knowledge and experience; weakness, because some OA members are perpetuating their pathorexia by striving to stay constitutionally underweight and receive unconditional support from fellow members for their oftentimes misguided efforts.

Nevertheless many of our clients have been greatly helped by OA. One who perhaps typifies the best outcome is Cathy, a housewife with two preschool children who believes that OA saved her marriage and maybe her life.

"I was always careful about my weight, but when I got pregnant with Jimmy, my second son, the doctor said I should gain some more weight to be on the safe side. That really panicked me, and of course I did just the opposite! . . . . Then when I was home from the hospital, all I could think about was food. There was nobody around, I felt really lonely, and somehow I started eating crackers and spitting them out. Once when I did that, I gagged and threw up. I was crying when it happened."

Within days of that experience, Cathy was eating crackers nonstop and pausing to throw up every twenty minutes. The behavior continued for three years and hardly changed even after she began psychotherapy.

She became sickly and depressed, and her marriage deteriorated. She rarely left home except to buy food. Finding plausible reasons for buying cartons of crackers became a troubling preoccupation. That, perhaps more than anything else, precipitated her decision to seek therapy.

Cathy contacted OA with our encouragement. Fortunately, her sponsor (the contact person assigned to new members) had had her own brush with bulimarexia. She knew how much support Cathy would need in the beginning. She helped Cathy substitute telephone calls for saltines—ten to fifteen separate calls a day in the first month. Gradually, Cathy was weaned from her dependency, and her life returned to normal. But OA is still important to her, both for the support she gets and for the help she now gives others.

During the 1970s, three organizations formed to help eating-disordered people: the National Association for Anorexia Nervosa and Associated Disorders, Inc. (ANAD); the American Anorexia/Bulimia Association (AABA); and the National Anorexia Aid Society (NAAS). They combined lay energy with professional input. We have listed the addresses and telephone numbers of these organizations at the end of the book. These groups helped publicize the fact that eating disorders are recognized and treatable phenomena that have been known for decades and have been treated successfully in hospitals and clinics.

These organizations also offered forums for parents and spouses of pathorexics—setting up meetings where these affected people could share their experiences. The anguish of watching helplessly or battling fruitlessly while a child or loved one was trapped in pathorexia no longer need be a lonely vigil.

Medical involvement with eating disorders has been available since they were diagnosed and named (a Doctor William Gull first used the term anorexia nervosa in London in 1874). But the treatments were not especially effective. Force feeding and punitive incarceration featured too prominently as therapy to give anorexics much assurance that they would be cared for with genuine sympathy. Though we can sense the frustration of hospital staffs confronted with patients who seemed bent on self-destruction, we know now that coercive techniques are generally counterproductive. They do nothing to promote long-term improvement and growth in self-respect.

In the nineteenth century and the first half of the twentieth, psychiatry often had to be content by offering diagnoses rather than treatment to the emotionally ill. Supportive care was its principal form of treatment. Psychoanalysis and some rival, but closely related, philosophies of personality had provided penetrating insights about the role of unconscious motives in determining human behavior. However, the application of these discoveries to patient care proved both very expensive and disappointing in its outcome.

Nevertheless, Freudian therapy dominated the profession. This resulted in anorexics (bulimics were still too rare to draw the attention of practical therapists) receiving a diagnostic straight jacket that labeled them afraid of adult sexuality. They were simply thought to be delaying maturation through deliberate malnutrition.

To be sure, many sensitive therapists were able, with care and understanding, to help patients recover from their disabling symptoms. Also, we should acknowledge the fact that sexual fears are often present in anorexia. But we now recognize the fact that self-starvation is a symptom that attaches itself to many emotional disorders and also to some physical ones.

People with eating disorders still have a reputation for yielding only to therapists with acute empathy and insight—keeping alive the self-fulfilling expectation that they are somehow special-problem people with a need for extra special attention.

The pioneering work in the 1950s and 1960s of some now famous therapists and researchers greatly expanded our knowledge of treatments for eating disorders. Hilde Bruch, Salvatore Minuchin, and Maria Selvini-Palazzoli, to name three, all helped identify the social context in which eating disorders occur. Their example shifted the treatment focus from the individual to the family. Few therapists today would consider working with an adolescent anorexic without having the parents, and maybe the siblings, in some form of treatment also.

Until the 1970s, bulimia and bulimarexia were generally assumed to be variants of anorexia nervosa. This was therapeutically unfortunate and served to suppress both the treatment options and the identification of patients. Much credit is due Marlene Boskind-White, who, as a psychologist at Cornell University in 1974, described and named bulimarexia.

She developed a successful therapy that addressed her patients' overly compliant femininity and broadened and strengthened their sense of identity. Her concepts revolutionized treatment goals and greatly increased the number of people seeking help.

Meanwhile, the physiology of eating and appetite has become better understood. Until recently, few people questioned the notion that we are free to choose how wide we want to be. It was presumed to be simply a matter of deciding how much fat to carry. We now know that this is false, but we are not sure just how false it is. Some of the variables that control appetite and adiposity have been identified, and we discuss them more thoroughly in Chapters 8 and 9.

Much more information about physiology and nutrition awaits clarification. Because we know that this knowledge will have a major impact on treatment goals and therapy, we can expect strategies to help pathorexics to evolve quickly in the light of new findings. So fresh is this field that a meeting in New York in November 1982 was billed as the "The First Annual Conference . . ." on the treatment of anorexia and bulimia. Another landmark was the publication in the Fall of 1981 of the first issue of the International Journal of Eating Disorders.

Now that there is widespread public awareness of pathorexia, the number of people seeking treatment increases daily. Many therapists are receiving orientation and training to meet this unprecedented demand for service, and eating disorder clinics are being organized at many psychiatric hospitals and mental health centers. This awareness will have many substantial and beneficial effects. First, the disorders will no longer be mysterious. Second, and very important, therapists and patients will discover that many people have brushes with pathorexia and recover—some spontaneously, others with brief treatment. This will allow people to gain a more accurate impression of how deeply involved they have become. It will also enable therapists to develop perspectives on treatment as they discover how psychological functioning relates to the severity of symptoms, giving them a selection of therapeutic goals to help patients progress toward healthy behaviors. And finally, it will enable therapists to develop preventive measures and techniques for early diagnosis that may limit the further spread of appetite disorders.

8
the physical causes of appetite disorders

"I'd rather throw up three times a day than
end up looking like my parents!"

The next two chapters provide a more complete explanation of the physical and psychological reasons why people develop pathorexic symptoms. We begin with the physical changes that occur and that cause a choice of behavior to develop into an addictive disease.

A rich, but by no means complete, body of knowledge has been gathered on the subject of appetite disorders. We have learned that there are six major factors that contribute to human appetite. They interact with each other in ways that are complex and unique to each individual. The factors are: heredity, fat deposits, metabolism, brain functions, learned behavior, and environment. When these forces are out of balance appetite disorders can develop.

Other factors that should be mentioned, though they are beyond the scope of this book to discuss, are medical and physical trauma. There are glandular and hormonal disorders and certain brain dysfunctions that affect both the appetite and metabolism. Many medications have an impact on appetite for people who are being treated for diseases unrelated to eating.

Some physical handicaps limit activity so much that obesity is almost inevitable. Certain emotional disorders, like depression, though only loosely associated with eating, may have a marked effect on appetite. Severe psychiatric disorders may also reveal themselves through pathorexic symptoms. When this is the case, bizarre eating behaviors are never the only signs of disorder. Other significant symptoms will also be evident.

Such disorders require intensive therapy, most often beginning with hospitalization, where careful diagnosis can be made. Treatment then addresses the underlying emotional disorder, not the external symptoms. The following case study is an example of a patient whose pathorexia was accompanied by a serious personality disorder.

MARLA

At 20 years of age, Marla had been an active bulimarexic for six years, during which time she had made two suicide attempts.

Her self-destructive impulses caused her to sabotage any friendships that might have threatened her isolation and made her perform physical acts of violence against herself. These included cutting her feet with broken glass and intentionally burning her lips, fingers, and arms with cigarettes. She selected certain sores and kept them open for months at a time by picking off scabs as they formed.

Marla vomited into a plastic bag in her bedroom wastebasket at least three times per day. During the purging, she turned up her radio to mask the sounds. Following the purging, she would sneak the bag into the bathroom at the far end of hall, empty it, and stealthily return it to her bedroom. Sometimes, other members of her large family kept the bathroom in constant use, forcing Marla to either hide the vomitus in her room or fling it from her second story window to escape detection.

It was after her second suicide attempt that Marla was brought to our attention. Her parents were totally unaware of Marla's many forms of self abuse and only sought therapy for their daughter at the insistence of her doctor.

We worked with Marla for over two years. Progress was very slow and not very steady, but she did improve. She was hospitalized twice when crises overcame her. She remained on medication throughout the entire treatment.

Marla's recovery required the joint efforts of psychologist, psychiatrists, and hospital personnel. Working alone, none of her therapists would have helped her.

If you suspect that other medical or psychiatric problems are contributing to an appetite disorder, seek competent professional help before you assume that the STEM program in Chapter 10 is sufficient to meet your needs.

Before we explain the underlying causes of appetite disorders, it may be helpful to review the nature of healthy appetite control. So far as we know, most people adjust their eating patterns to meet their needs with relatively little personal effort. Physical and psychological forces operate smoothly and effectively in a cooperative fashion.

While food intake does not precisely match energy expenditure, a balance is maintained such that physical appearances or sizes in clothes do not alter appreciably. In addition, the balance occurs at a size and weight that allows the optimal physical health to be achieved.

Like everyone else, healthy eaters experience the temptation to overindulge and overeat from time to time. However, for reasons that are not at all well understood, it takes little effort on their part to regain a healthy equilibrium. It is most probable that healthy people routinely eat more than is nutritionally necessary. Their metabolisms adjust to the excess to prevent unneeded weight gain. This ability to compensate is lost by people who force upon themselves a regimen of semi-starvation in order to alter their shape. The failure of these normal regulating mechanisms is the principal cause of pathorexia.

The Anatomy of Appetite

Heredity Part of the biological inheritance we receive from our parents is a set of genes that will decide for us the basic size and shape of our bones, muscles, and fat deposits. The circumstances in which we grow up may modify these proportions, but there are limits to the possible changes. To some degree, we all resemble our parents. Characteristic facial features and body builds typically identify family members in several generations. Similarly, the tendency to be heavy runs in families. It has been shown that there is an 80 percent chance that the children of obese parents will also become obese.

We vividly recall a client who told us about his Jewish grandmother who had been hidden in a cellar in France during World War II. Despite the fact that she had survived on minimal rations for almost three years, she was still quite rounded when she emerged. This proved to be something of an embarrassment for her at the time, just as the same genetic tendency to obesity embarrassed her grandson, albeit in totally different and far less pressured circumstances.

In this century, an American psychologist, William Sheldon, compiled the most comprehensive and scientific information on body types to date.

Based on an analysis of thousands of specially posed photographs, he derived a three-part classification of body types. He named them *endomorphs*, *mesomorphs*, and *ectomorphs*, referring to tendencies to be soft and round, square and muscular, or thin and skeletal. Sheldon showed that every body has a blend of these traits in a measurable degree.

He devised a complex but reliable formula for labeling body types and recorded them on three seven-point scales. Thus, a completely endomorphic person was scored 7-1-1, a perfect mesomorph 1-7-1, and a total ectomorph 1-1-7. A completely balanced body was rated 4-4-4.

Sheldon claimed that the body type is an unalterable inheritance and demonstrated that his system of measurement produced the same scores for people who were tested repeatedly over several years, even after weight changes of as much as 100 pounds.

Other researchers disputed his conviction that body type is a stable trait. In a famous study of malnutrition in which volunteers underwent six months of semi-starvation, scientist Ancel Keys claimed that his subjects had become more ectomorphic. But two years later, they had all returned to their original shapes. This demonstrated most effectively that although shape can be modified, only continued undernutrition will maintain unnatural thinness.

Another scientist, Ethan Allen Sims, overfed volunteers to induce weight gain. His results led to similar conclusions. Weight gain proved hard to achieve and was only temporary. A return to an unforced diet was followed by the loss of the excess weight in almost all of his subjects.

Sheldon went on to describe characteristic temperaments for the various body types he had identified. He repeatedly referred to the ectomorph's love of food, often with affection. He wrote of their "deep joy in eating," and observed that for endomorphs, "The soul has its seat in the splendid gut." He showed a refreshing acceptance of both natural and acquired fat by referring to weight gain as "blossoming."

Because Sheldon used complex calculations to determine body type, it is not practical to duplicate his techniques—nor is it necessary. The short questionnaire that follows will help you decide whether you are predominantly one type, whether you are a mixture of two principal types, or whether you are a balanced mid-ranger who has some features of all three body types. The items are based upon characteristics that are associated with each body type.

Body Type Questionnaire

Score one point for every characteristic which is often true of you. You may check more than one item in some rows—this means that you have the attributes of two or more body types.

Endomorphy		*Mesomorphy*		*Ectomorphy*	
Relaxed posture and movement	(✓)	Assertive posture and movement	( )	Restrained posture and movement	( )
Love of physical comfort	( )	Love of physical adventure	( )	Secretive emotions, self consciousness	( )
Love of eating	( )	Love of activity	( )	Love of quiet	( )
Love of social activities	( )	Pleasure in competition	( )	Resistance to habit and routine	( )
Love of approval and affection	( )	Delight in gaining authority	( )	Slow physical maturation	( )
Need for people when troubled	( )	Need for action when troubled	( )	Need for solitude when troubled	( )
Relaxed, friendly with alcohol	( )	Noisy, aggressive when drinking	( )	Distaste, avoidance of alcohol	( )
Soft, rounded physique	( )	Thick, muscular underlayer	( )	Slender, bony frame	( )
TOTAL ENDOMORPHY	( )	TOTAL MESOMORPHY	( )	TOTAL ECTOMORPHY	( )

In addition to developing his technique for classifying body types, Sheldon and his co-workers studied the natural changes in weight and shape that accompany aging. They discovered that certain body types maintain a stable weight throughout adult life, while those people with significant endomorphy gradually fill out until late middle-age when they are apt to shrink a little.

The amount of normal change is predictable and varies with the degree of endomorphy.

These findings are hardly surprising. They conform precisely with our everyday experience that some people get rounder as they get older while others do not. Only the dictates of fashion and unrealistically dogmatic height and weight charts that make no allowance for age or body type conflict with Sheldon's data. Unfortunately, most people pay more attention to fashion than to physiology and, as a consequence, put themselves in a higher risk category for appetite disorders.

It has been our impression that women with significant mesomorphism are especially vulnerable to appetite disorders. They tend to have squarish frames with an appropriate overlay of fat. Young women with this heritage usually have had an easy time being social and adapting to developmental tasks as children, but they begin to feel uncomfortable about their shape in high school.

They view the need to trim off 15 to 20 pounds as a modest challenge and often confront it by crash dieting. Their bodies' stubborn resistance to being starved comes as a shock to them, and their subsequent development of pathorexic symptoms may be their first experience with failure. Being praised and rewarded for becoming more attractive while they are aware that they are not quite well creates a painful and confusing dilemma. The following story from our files is a good illustration.

JUNE

June was 16, a high-school junior, when she developed pathorexia. Although she was an excellent student with disciplined study habits, June had distinguished herself most through her athletic prowess. On three varsity teams and captain of the soccer team, she was universally regarded as a leader. Her consistent patience and good humor resulted in many demands on her time for coaching and supervision. A joy to her parents and an honored student, June seemed to have the world on a string.

Problems began when June decided that it was important that she be invited to her school's Winter Ball. She was dismayed to find that a couple of hints she had dropped were not acted upon, and much to her chagrin, she was faced with the choice of not attending or going with a girlfriend.

June was not about to accept second best. She stayed home, brooded over what had gone wrong, and stared at herself in the mirror in a mood tinged with anger and despair.

Suddenly, her athlete's body seemed all wrong. Her broad shoulders and muscled calves and thighs were, she decided, the cause of her rejection.

Immediately, June exercised her customary determination toward a new goal. In three weeks, she lost 15 pounds, putting herself three pounds below the minimum weight for her height, according to a table she found in a women's magazine.

The next shock for June was the discovery that maintaining her new weight was more difficult than achieving it. Her favorite study corner in the kitchen became a place where unmanagable temptations to eat swept over her. While she remained proud of her novel, but barely perceptible, slimness, she was also plagued with sharp mood swings and lost ground in academics and athletics.

June's parents quickly became involved. Mystified by her upset emotions and then disturbed by her change in behavior, they nevertheless applauded her decision to lose weight, because they were perpetually restraining their own appetites. Their first hint that something was seriously amiss came the night they returned home late to find the refrigerator bare of all food and the pantry bereft of bread, cereal, crackers and cookies. This was the first and worst in a series of solitary raids that June made on the family food supply. These raids resulted in a marked rift with her parents.

June's mother tried a variety of sensible meal plans to help June cope with her cravings, but each failed. After eight weeks of continued pain and tension, June's mother sent her to a dietitian. June's determination to stay underweight was not approved by the dietitian, who recommended more food and referred her to us for psychological help.

June had great difficulty coming to terms with the idea that her muscular body was a characteristic she could not abandon simply because it was no longer fashionable. In order to accept her figure, she found it necessary to question and revise many other aspects of her identity that she had previously taken for granted. When last we saw her, she had compromised by gaining back between eight and ten of the lost pounds and had settled for an appetite she could control most of the time. She had chosen nutrition for her college major.

Sheldon's work implies that beautiful people with well balanced physiques are blessed with beautiful genes. Fortunately we do not have to be "beautiful" to be healthy. For many of us, optimal physical and mental health will not mean that we are necessarily good looking. It is all too likely that our natural allotment of fatty tissues will lie outside the current norms for beauty, both in quantity and distribution.

Nevertheless, physical and emotional health is a winning combination, making a striking appearance irrelevant. True happiness is never solely dependent upon the shape of our bodies. When an inherently plain person becomes convinced that the route to greater popularity and contentment lies in changing fat distribution through diet programs, the potential for pathorexia is created.

The vast majority of us inherit proportions that are comfortably within the limits for good health. Occasionally, a genetic predisposition towards unhealthy fatness may occur. At present, our knowledge of this possibility is still limited. We do not know how often such defects appear.

From animal experiments, we know that obesity can be bred into a strain of laboratory mice until all offspring develop the condition, but the chance occurrence of obesity in animals is rare. It is possible that in humans, congenitally determined obesity occurs more often.

Adiposity This is the second closely related factor in the control of appetite: the number of fat cells in the body. Normal fat cells are primarily laid down during childhood and adolescence. It is believed that how these cells are formed is determined in part by genetics and in part by nutrition. It is also thought that, by and large, the total number of fat cells cannot be reduced after they have formed, though an unhealthy excess may form during major weight gain.

We conclude from this that feeding patterns in the early years of our lives and in adolescence have a lifelong influence on our shape and, indirectly, on our appetites. If as a child we were indulged with a rich and plentiful supply of food, we may have built up a burden of fat cells that will plague us until death.

The number of fat cells we possess is not the only variable associated with adiposity. Their size is also important. The principal purpose of these cells is as a readily available source of energy for the body. They constitute our fuel supply, and, as such, they are continually being built up or drawn upon. They function by varying in size rather than number.

In healthy people, these variations in size are too subtle to be detectable, but in pathorexics this is not so. Because their ineffective appetite control systems cause them to overeat, pathorexics' fat cells are subject to major inflation. After reaching a maximum diameter, more cells may form if excess intake continues.

The Guinness Book of World Records reports about people weighing as much as 1,000 pounds and being crushed by their own weight. Photographs of such people show clearly that their excess weight is in the form of fat. With dieting, those fat cells could be reduced practically to invisibility, but they would not be destroyed, and they would not disappear.

We do not know how much direct effect the size of our fat cells has on our appetite. It is probable that feedback circuits exist that serve to increase hunger as the cells shrink, in order that our energy reserves do not become too depleted. Of course, if we have too many cells to begin with, that alarm system is going to sound too soon, and the struggle to reduce to average weight and then maintain it will be that much more difficult.

There are also indications that the rate of growth of fat cells is related to their size. In other words, the larger they are, the greater is their tendency to further enlarge. To the extent that this is true, it makes it doubly hard for the overweight person to halt continued weight gain.

In addition to the physical effects, excess adiposity has a powerful psychological impact. Sometimes it strengthens the resolve to lose weight, but all too often it fosters a depressed mood that typically leads to overeating and more weight gain.

Whether an internal monitoring function exists or whether fat cells have only a psychological effect on appetite, their presence in excess creates a form of obesity that is especially resistant to weight-reducing programs. The condition is most common in people who become heavy in childhood or adolescence. Many such endomorphic people are quite at home with their soft, round physiques, and they enjoy temperaments that accord with their appearance. Research indicates that their mental health and self-respect fall within normal limits, and they live full and happy lives. They never expect to be slim, and they have always been aware that their above average weight can inflate into obesity when they give in to their overactive appetites.

Others, however, never accept their bodies. They fight a constant battle with themselves, and their sense of wellbeing is inversely proportional to their weight.

LAURA

Laura may have been regarded as a "pleasantly plump" baby. Certainly, her early photographs would indicate the appropriateness of that label. However, by the age of five, she looked like a rather typical little girl complete with skinny legs and knobby knees.

She has early memories of her mother telling her, after she had had enough to eat, that she must be careful not to end up looking like Aunt Susan (mother's overweight sister), who mother never failed to ridicule. Laura remembers leaving the table hungry but receiving praise when she mentioned not having satisfied her appetite.

During Laura's pre-teen and teenage years, her mother and father commented daily on her adorable and sweet appearance. When Laura showed interest in what her folks considered to be *extra* food, her parents always told her not to ruin her figure and complexion. Dad would then suggest that "his ladies go on a little shopping spree." The family was well-off financially, and buying new outfits was a well-established female role, second only to cooking and laundering.

Laura recalls *always* feeling a bit hungry but feeling very beautiful and refined in her expensive clothes. She would, in fact, binge on clothing, often buying outfits for which she had no use but in which she thought she looked good. Today, many of them remain unworn in her closet.

At 25, Laura married and within a few months became pregnant. Knowledge of her impending weight gain seemed to give Laura permission to eat, and eat she did. Before the first trimester was over, her physician expressed concern about her excessive weight gain. Laura denied the seriousness of this warning and continued to eat all she wanted of everything. The weight gain continued, the warnings continued, the ignoring continued. Finally, Laura developed toxemia, and the delivery of her baby had to be induced one month early.

Following the birth of her child, Laura was able to shed only 5 of the 65 pounds she had gained. In reviewing her case history, it appears that a foundation of extra adipose cells developed during infancy and remained dormant because of Laura's strict restraint of food intake until she became pregnant. Once she gave up control of her appetite, the weight gain was rapid.

Laura has remained at least 40 pounds over her pre-pregnancy weight, and, though she is not happy with her appearance, there have been no further medical complications.

Metabolism and Appetite As we might reasonably expect, the digestive system and the brain both have a large role in controlling appetite and eating. Sensory organs in the stomach, the intestine, and the liver monitor the system's current need for food and help regulate eating behavior on an hour to hour basis.

The brain's role is probably more tuned toward long-term maintenance of the whole organism, deciding when there is a need to increase or decrease fat stores. The brain is possibly a nutritional monitor also, subtly directing us to consume needed quantities of protein, vitamins, and minerals to maintain optimal health and functioning.

The stomach swells and shrinks in the course of its work and secretes various gastric juices during that cycle. Normal individuals seem able to sense these and other physiological variations, such as blood sugar level, and are able to translate them into the discomfort of hunger and the pleasure of satiety. It is likely that healthy persons pick up these subtle cues and the obvious, more visual ones—like the amount of food that has disappeared from the plate—and stop eating to avoid the unpleasant consequences of overindulgence.

Pathorexics seem to lack this ability. Experiments have shown that their experience of hunger has less connection with the amount of food present in their stomachs than is the case with normal persons. They continue eating, even though their stomachs are full. Conversely, many pathorexics fail to recognize their need for food and, in its absence, can go for much longer periods of time than normal people without feeling hungry.

Unfortunately, this attribute is more than cancelled out by their inability to refrain from eating when food is present. Experiments have shown them to be significantly more aware of and aroused by the sight or smell of food. A physiological reason for this has been shown to be their tendency to secrete the gastric hormone *insulin* when they see, smell, or think about attractive foods. Insulin, which is needed for absorption of food, triggers appetite, and excess insulin not only arouses appetite but also maintains it when the stomach is full. This leads many pathorexics to continue eating even though they feel physically uncomfortable and know they would be wise to stop.

This phenomenon has been measured by comparing the response to sugar by pathorexics and normals. Healthy people tire of the taste of sugar as their stomachs fill, but pathorexics are happy to continue eating sweets and desserts for much longer periods of time. These differences go a long way to explain the familiar conflict between appetite and willpower that pathorexics experience each time they have more food available than they need.

The hormone imbalances that are associated with too much insulin are complex and vary greatly between individuals. They also have widely varying effects on energy, mood, hunger, and other physical sensations. The craving for food late at night, for example, may well be triggered physiologically. So, too, may be desires for unusual foods, loss of ability to concentrate, mood swings, sweating, dizziness, and other minor upsets. The relationships between nutrition and a sense of well-being are only just being unravelled.

An unresolved question about hyperinsulinism, as this condition is called, concerns the extent to which it may be induced by dieting. It is well known that the body reacts defensively to sharp reductions in food supply. Metabolism slows down, tissue replacement is deferred, and both fat and lean mass is sacrificed. In order to promote eating behavior, the appetite may quicken.

When dieters refeed, their bodies rebuild fat stores first and often compensate for the trauma of dieting by laying down more fat than was lost. Hence, the common dilemma of quick weight loss being followed by a regain of weight to a new and higher total weight. Hyperinsulinism is the body's response to unhealthy weight loss and may intensify with each round of dieting and weight gain.

Our experience indicates that for some people a quick loss of as little as six pounds may trigger pathorexia. Thus, the treadmill of chronic dieting and perpetual hunger in the presence of food begins with the seemingly innocent first step of trimming a few pounds for cosmetic effect.

Appetite and the Brain The brain's role in controlling appetite can be considered under two categories: instinctual behaviors that happen without thought and psychological behaviors where we act according to how we feel or how we believe we must. It is the former that we discuss in this section. Psychological factors are considered in the next chapter.

The part of the brain that influences appetite seems to be located near the *hypothalamus*, which is a primitive organ that we share with much older and less evolved animals, including reptiles and fish. It is here that the mechanism that triggers insulin release is located. Because of the limitations on experimenting with live humans, much of our knowledge of hypothalamic appetite control is derived from work with animals, especially rats and mice.

It has been found that this nerve center is very important to rodents and exerts major control over their appetite and adiposity. Normal adult rats generally maintain their weight within close limits. However, when tiny cuts are made in areas of the brain close to the hypothalamus, the animals make drastic changes in their diets. Depending upon the locations of these lesions, they may gain weight or lose it.

After a certain amount of weight change has occurred, the rats actively work to maintain their new size. They counteract, to the extent they can, any forced feeding or fasting their experimenters impose upon them. Rats that have become obese seek to stay fat. Rats with depleted fat stores resist attempts to restore them to a more healthy weight.

The implications of this research for humans is still being explored, but it raises some interesting speculations. It is possible, for example, that *normal weight*, while being, in part, genetically determined, may also be governed by mechanisms in the brain that could sometimes operate without regard to overall health.

This could mean that some persons who already regard themselves as unhealthy, overweight people are being prompted, instinctually, to gain more weight, or to reach a higher weight, or *set-point*, that is determined by their hypothalamus. An excellent discussion of this subject can be found in the book *The Dieter's Dilemma* that is listed in the suggested readings at the end of this book.

On the other hand, some anorexics may have brain dysfunctions that sharply reduce their appetites. Indirect evidence exists that suggests that some types of physical abnormalities contribute to some forms of appetite disorder. Certain drugs that alter brain chemistry provoke and inhibit appetite and cause temporary weight changes. This raises the distinct possibility that medications may be developed that can alter appetite and restore normal eating patterns.

Although the hypothalamus plays a major part in appetite control, it has a far less significant role in humans than in rats and other experimental animals. The human brain is dominated by a massive *cerebral cortex* that other animals lack. The cortex is our cognitive center. It is where we store information and learn to make decisions based on knowledge rather than instinct. Our cortex gives us the power to interfere, modify, and override many of the instinctual patterns of the lower brain centers. In the long run, what we *learn* to do has more influence on our behavior than what we are born *able* to do. It is most important to always remember that no matter how deeply enmeshed in appetite disorder a person may be, the road to recovery still lies chiefly in learning new ways to look at life, ways that allow for growth and understanding.

Another way that the brain contributes to pathorexia is by creating a sense of calm following vomiting by releasing the body's natural pain killers called *endorphins*. Endorphins are substances chemically related to morphine that are potent pain killers. Unfortunately, like morphine and heroin, endorphins create an addiction. Bulimarexics become as addicted to purging as narcotic addicts are to heroin.

While we have not yet been able to study endorphin levels following vomiting, they have been detected after other physical stresses have been imposed on the subject. The observed responses are so akin to the accounts we have heard from numerous compulsive vomiters, that we are confident that this is another physical cause of bulimarexia. We close this chapter with a case history that illustrates the phenomenon of auto-addiction.

Pam was a patient we treated on and off for two years. She returned after 6 months without therapy, saying that although her life has improved dramatically and she no longer felt prompted to binge and purge because of stress, she had experienced an irresistible urge to resume vomiting. Discussion lead us to conclude that Pam had become addicted to the feeling of calm that followed the purge, a calm that she said was just like the *runner's high* she used to experience when she ran several miles a day. She noted, too, that purging had replaced exercise in her life, a change that puzzled and troubled her. By recognizing that her addiction had shifted from a psychological to a physiological pressure, Pam had the strength to reduce the frequency of her purges, although she continues to find them a source of tranquility that she calls on from time to time.

9
the psychology
of appetite disorders

"Every time Jack 'worked late at the office'
I'd empty the refrigerator and then head for the bathroom."

Human beings, like all living organisms, seek food spontaneously and respond physically to the sight or smell of food. Unlike other organisms, however, humans do not have simple, inborn characteristics that set limits to that search and response.

As soon as we are born, our parents and other caretakers move to socialize our food seeking behavior. In the process, they distort the relationship between our nutritional needs and our appetite.

In the beginning, this is all done for our own good, of course. The process gets underway the first time our mother offers us affection instead of food when we are hungry. From then on the interference never ends. First comes the scheduling of meals to meet the needs of the family. Later there is encouragement to eat all the food prepared. Then there is good food versus poor food, treats and luxuries, the starving children in Asia, feasts, stories of famines, waiting until everyone is served, never taking the biggest slice, permissible snacks and forbidden snacks, watching one's weight, and getting a good breakfast every morning.

There is guidance and manipulation. There are good examples and bad examples. There is education, and there is propaganda.

The only thing there never is, is silence.

Although most of our attitudes toward food and eating are formed in childhood, some major changes may occur at the second threshold of life, entry to adulthood. This is a time when the influence of peers may shift behavior from the established family patterns.

A common example that occurs at this time is learning to vomit to avoid the consequences of overindulgence in alcohol.

College students living in dormitories often have to deal with dining hall rules that encourage food abuse. Bingeing, hoarding, and stealing often begin as ways to cope with rushed meals, kitchens closing early, and inadequate quantities of quality food. Poorly prepared food can lead to reliance on candy or desserts to compensate for inedible cafeteria meals. Weight gain from too much starchy food may lead to imprudent dieting and self-starvation.

Young people who move into their own living quarters and cook for themselves for the first time also have a tendency to take short cuts with food preparation. In a susceptible individual, these changes can set in motion a drift into pathorexia.

These processes are both social and psychological. The social components are the inputs from society to the individual and the responses to society by the individual. The psychological components are the interactions between the individual's genetic endowment and the parental and social outputs.

The prospect of ever truly disentangling the genetic from the social inputs, so that the unique contribution of each can be identified, is very remote, but we do know that constitutional differences affect what we learn and how we respond.

Inherent psychological variables surely cause some people to favor the parental injunction to "eat what is served" over the conflicting injunction "don't gain weight!" Others will adopt the reverse position. Also, the degree to which the stomach and the brain effect behavior in the face of social attempts to override these injunctions must vary from person to person.

So each one of us grows up in a unique confusion of conflicting and contradictory messages about the primary sustaining force in life—our appetite.

Because of the physical necessity that we eat every few hours, it is likely that no aspect of our growth and maturation receives as much attention as our eating patterns. We are taught to associate food with a host of connected attitudes and values, some of them clearly detrimental to our health.

For example, most of us learn to appreciate the taste of candy, which is nutritionally poor but frequently associated with affection, and to recoil from nourishing vegetables because they are so often presented with coercion. In early childhood, we develop a hierarchy of preference for various foods, and our parents find it difficult to resist the temptation to control our behavior by offering and withdrawing favored goodies.

The relationship between flavor and appetite is fascinating. We are learning rapidly, but still have far to go. Flavor is the most intimate environmental factor affecting appetite and probably has important consequences for health. We know that humans and animals have a powerful tendency to prefer sweeter, and therefore riper, fruits and vegetables, and this mechanism has obvious survival value.

The relatively recent development (i.e. since the Industrial Revolution of the 18th century) of techniques for the inexpensive refining and manufacture of sugar has led to the growth of huge companies dedicated to its production and has greatly increased the sweetness of our diets. Human biology has not changed to compensate for this environmental revolution. We still prefer sweet food, though this is more likely to be hazardous than healthy.

Some people sense their personalities change dramatically, and for the worse, when they consume sugar. A patient told us this:

> "When I get into sugars I'm a Jekyll and Hyde. I 'numb out.' I'm totally out of touch with my feelings, but I'll rationalize anything to keep eating. I'll even think I need to gain weight! I can see it in my mother, too. When she's on sugar, I can't trust her with information. She twists and distorts anything I say."

A similar situation exists with respect to fats. These cheap, high-caloric substances have little flavor themselves, but when they are added to other foods, they greatly enhance their palatability. Because they are relatively inexpensive, they are used in vast quantities by the food industry.

Many experts sense that these changes have caused a massive deformation in the world's nutrition. Others find no reason for concern. As we await harder information, it is wise to monitor and restrain our personal consumption of sugar, sweeteners, and fats, and we should seek to rediscover the subtler flavors of less processed foods.

The net result of this barrage of manipulation—familial, social, and commercial—is to create for each of us an artificial structure of needs and motivations, when dealing with food and eating.

Although every one of us is different, some trends and tendencies can be applied to all. Surely the most widespread characteristic of all is the linkage of eating and affection. It is a simple human pleasure to feed those whom we love. When our own search for love is inhibited, many of us find comfort by substituting food just as, if our search for food were frustrated, we would surely find comfort in the closeness and warmth of love.

Psychoanalysts have developed comprehensive explanations of human behavior based upon the interaction between affection and feeding in the first months of a baby's life. Anyone who has spent time with weight-control programs is aware that, while almost all food is hard to resist, Grandma's cake and Mom's apple pie are the treats that are most difficult to refuse. The psychology of infancy finds an echo and a reenactment in every decade of our lives.

It may be that people who experience much uncertainty or insecurity as children are especially susceptible to appetite disorders. Animal studies have shown that unpredictable feeding schedules create increased appetites in young rats, and there is clinical evidence suggesting parallels with children from troubled families.

> We are reminded of a sixteen-year-old girl, Beth, an only child, whose parents had divorced and remarried and had joint custody of their daughter. After several months of treatment, Beth came to recognize the fact that she felt responsible for keeping all four parents and stepparents happy. The stress generated by this impossible responsibility precipitated her illness. Beth felt that the concern generated by the illness kept her stepfamilies cooperating, and it also allowed her to avenge the hurt she felt when her parents divorced. Later, she realized that her folks had made many problems worse because, although they worried about her, they blamed each other for the situation.

> Beth gradually separated herself from her parents' conflicting expectations. Counseling helped her to recognize the fact that her anger was misplaced, and, as stress was lifted, her pathorexia subsided. As her health improved, her parents no longer needed to be in such close contact with each other. The vicious cycle of conflicts reinforcing the symptoms was reversed. When the pressure was relieved, Beth learned how to appreciate her extended family, instead of feeling oppressed by it.

One important human attribute is our ability to find substitute satisfactions when our primary needs cannot be met. Most of these compensatory mechanisms work to our advantage: for example, when a child who loses a parent succeeds in bonding with another supportive adult. Sometimes, however, these substitutions are symbolic instead of real. The analogy between sports and warfare is a commonly recognized and approved transformation.

Occasionally substitution works against us. Clinical psychologists often find that an emotional disorder becomes more difficult to treat when forbidden or inhibited thoughts or behaviors are acted out through acceptable but inappropriate symbolic gestures.

The acts of eating, fasting, and vomiting can easily become symbols of affection, control, and anger. If these emotional associations are powerful and compelling and the same emotions do not have a normal outlet in daily life, the symbolic acts may become addictive behaviors. Because these behaviors are only symbolic, they never truly work to resolve problems. Nevertheless, they do provide a modest sense of relief and, as such, get repeated over and over in a fruitless quest for peace.

Anorexics are especially prone to entrapment in these fantasies. Eating and fat become symbols of weakness, while fasting is equated with power.

> Ruth, while well on the way to recovery from bulimarexia, had a relapse into anorexia when she fell in love. Believing that she had to avoid being "just another ordinary person," Ruth became convinced that she would be able to stop her boyfriend from leaving if she quit eating lunch.

> Another anorexic having romantic difficulties invited her boyfriend to dinner with the family. When he was late in arriving, she turned to her mother and said coolly, "If he doesn't come, I'm not eating this food!"

Another almost universal custom is the inclusion of food in ceremonies of celebration. Most of us feel a strong desire to use food to enhance any pleasurable occasion. While Thanksgiving dinner has a clear historical connection with the harvest, other everyday situations have become inappropriately food-related: football on television prompts us to break out beer and pretzels; movies are not the same without popcorn; a coffee break tends to be enriched with a doughnut.

These and many similar situations can infiltrate our lives to the point where we no longer regard the associated foods as treats but as essential accompaniments to the occasions. Without them, the events would no longer be enjoyable. When food consumption becomes linked in this way to between-meal activities, the influence of physical cues that signal satisfaction are diminished. Our appetites get triggered by our environment instead of our bodies.

A widespread but hazardous behavior pattern is the willingness to let other people decide for us what and how much we should eat. As a mark of respect to a host, we naturally try to eat what is offered for a meal or refreshment. Meanwhile, our host, out of respect for us, tries to serve enough food to make sure no one remains hungry. All too often the net result is that significant overfeeding takes place. This often sets a standard for subsequent socializing.

In addition, twentieth-century abundance has created a situation in which many families prepare, daily, as lavish a table as in the past would have been reserved for feasts. The consequence is that most of us have established a level of richness and quantity in food service that far exceeds what is needed for good health.

For many people, affluence has lead to the assumption that hunger can and should be banished. Indeed, there are people who cannot remember when last they felt hungry. From there, it is a short step to becoming afraid of being hungry. Such people embrace overeating and perhaps other forms of pathorexia as their salvation from the normal, invigorating experience of hunger that is a thrice daily event for healthy persons.

The common thread through these examples of the social pressures to alter our eating behaviors is that they all serve to separate our appetites from our nutritional needs. (Indeed this is very often a conscious goal: the host who can overcome a guest's reluctance to accept a second helping scores a social victory.) In this way, our appetites are redirected, and we lose touch with our personal needs while learning to substitute social customs. This often leads to excessive eating, obesity, an unfashionable appearance, and the disapproval of the very persons who previously encouraged the overindulgence.

Girls and women seem especially vulnerable to this cruel irony because they are raised to be sensitive to others' needs. As children, in order to conform to parental wishes, they allow themselves to be overfed, only to discover as teenagers that they are criticized for being fat.

Many women diet themselves thin as they search for a husband and marry at the lightest weight of their adult lives. Only later do they permit their natural size and shape to emerge. Such women are victims of a double bind in which they sense that people close to them are giving them two contradictory messages: "Come eat with us," and, "Be slim and lovely."

This conflict always causes a loss of self-respect for persons programmed to please others. The misery is particularly intense in adolescence if there is a significant failure to arouse the interest of potential lovers. As making friends and attracting sexual partners is a hugely important aspect of life for young adults, some of them find themselves totally consumed with this project.

Again, women are especially prone to problems because they know that their appearance is a vital part in the dating game. If they lack social confidence, they often blame their figures for their disappointments, ignoring the fact that many of their equally imperfect peers pair off with ease. Bulimarexia often develops as a consequence of this crisis. It is initially experienced as a blessed relief from the pressures of the double bind—being able to eat all that is served yet still maintaining or losing weight.

But the cycle of overeating and vomiting induces its own varieties of psychic pain. Victims soon feel alone and trapped in a disgusting but inescapable behavior pattern that takes over their lives. A facade of contentment often conceals a suicidal inner despair. Now, when a chance for sexual relations occurs, it is likely to be sabotaged, pursued mechanically and lovelessly, or an uncaring partner is chosen because a sense of unworthiness pervades the whole personality. Bulimarexia is a vicious and punishing emotional disorder.

JUDY

Judy came to see us at age 20 for help with a very severe case of bulimarexia. She had been diagnosed as anorexic in high school and had seen several therapists, although she had never been hospitalized. She reported years of "cold war" with her father, who is a graduate of a prestigious eastern business school. The cold war usually took the form of the father being "disappointed," and Judy usually retreated to her mother in the kitchen. She and her mother shared quiet criticisms of her Dad, but neither ever spoke up to him.

Judy continued to see her parents regularly even after she had moved out of the house. She reported still feeling like an object to them, being walked around and "shown" to people at cocktail parties and other social occasions. Typically, her folks would describe how Judy was going to put herself through law school by doing television commercials—"She's so pretty, she already has offers," they would exaggerate.

Despite Judy's recognition of her non-person status in their eyes, she would say, "But what right do I have to get angry with them? They are my parents and they really only want what's best for me. My father doesn't mean to be harsh. He just wants to see me live up to my full potential." Meanwhile the secret bingeing and vomiting continued.

Judy gradually improved. First she had to realize how unrealistic her parents' goals were for her. Then she had to realize that she had a right to set her *own* goals—to decide what she wanted for herself. Eventually, her vomiting occurred only once or twice a week. At this point, she decided to move far away and change her career. This broke her dependency on her father's opinions and allowed Judy to set herself free. When we last heard from her, she was doing well and felt truly happy for the first time she could remember. Her relationship with her parents was still difficult, but Judy was reconciled to it being somewhat forced until they became accustomed to her emancipation.

There are many more psychosocial and environmental reasons concerning why pathorexia develops than we have considered in this section. Many are commonplace experiences, and we could easily cite examples that are caused by economic factors, aesthetic issues, dietary customs, sex role conflicts and business practices, to name only a few of the widely divergent themes that can be linked to upsets in appetite which lead to pathorexia. An exhaustive accounting of the environmental aspects that cause pathorexia will never be realized because variations evolve continuously. It is doubtful one could even track down all the factors in a single individual's life.

For this reason, the treatment of appetite disorder must focus very clearly on the personal story of each victim.

10
stem
a program for recovery

"Recovery meant discovering myself—having an identity that stemmed from what I am, not from what I ate, or even how I looked."

We have described pathorexia as a disorder that upsets a complex equilibrium of genetic, physiological, psychological, and environmental factors. We have shown that pathorexia arises in a variety of ways, by pressures operating on any or all of these aspects of a person's being. Now, as we turn to techniques for combating pathorexia, it is essential to keep in mind how individual the disease is and how varied its causes are.

In proposing a program for the relief of pathorexia, it is wise to adopt an appropriate humility with regard to recovery. The professional and popular literature is littered with hundreds of proposals that have failed: programs that promise to banish anguish, diets and exercises to sculpt fresh bodies from old flesh, pills and medications to quell appetite forever, and strange garments and machines to melt fat in minutes. All appear and disappear in an endless cycle.

No mass-circulation women's magazine lets an issue go out without publishing a weight loss program of some kind. We can draw a number of conclusions from this:

1. Diets and exercise programs sell magazines and books.

2. Even though it is never correctly identified, appetite disorder must be a widespread affliction.

3. Each program must help some people in some way, thus giving it credibility, but no program works for most people—if one did it would be universally acclaimed, and deservedly so.

As you know, pathorexia is a stubborn disorder. It involves the entire organism—physiologically and psychologically. For most victims, it causes major disruptions in their personal and social lives, and it gnaws continually at their self-respect. To overcome it, we are about to propose another diet and exercise program. We know that it had better have some unique features if it is not about to share the same fate as all the others. This program is indeed unique, and this is why:

1. We address appetite first, eating second, and appearance and weight last.

2. We promise no short term benefits.

3. We challenge you to work out your own program and leave you with complete control of your individual plan.

4. We encourage you to incorporate a changing repertoire of new ideas taken from any source, provided that you are confident that they are right for you.

It is called the STEM plan. STEM is an acronym for Strategy Tactics Education & Monitoring.

The STEM plan is a guide to the big solution. If you use it, it will change your life. Here is how it works.

The four parts of the STEM plan form an interrelated set of activities that reinforce each other in the battle against pathorexia. Strategy refers to a basic orientation toward healthful living. Tactics are the daily activities that spring from and accomplish that plan. Education is keeping informed about matters that are relevant to your plan. And Monitoring is recording plans and keeping track of progress. Here is an example of how a very small STEM plan might work.

> GOAL: To improve heart and lung functioning and to lose some
> excess weight.

STRATEGY: Investigate local opportunities for dance and exercise classes or indoor sports programs, and make friends with people in those activities.

TACTICS: Rearrange your daily schedule to create time to sample the options available. Join the most attractive programs. Then seek occasions to be social with fellow members.

EDUCATION: Check with a physician or other qualified person to discover how much exercise will be wise, given your present physical condition.

MONITORING: Keep a diary listing your plans, your progress, your impressions, and your pulse, respiration, and weight.

So that is it in a nutshell. Now let us consider the parts in more detail.

Program Goal

The STEM concept can be used to pursue a variety of goals, so it is vital that you have a clear sense of what you want to accomplish. As you know, there are a variety of appetite disorders. The type of pathorexia you suffer from will influence how you treat it. Personal diagnosis becomes the first step in the program.

What sort of person are you, and what sort of eating disorder do you have? Are you an endomorph or a mesomorph striving to look like an emaciated ectomorph? Are you comfortable with the knowledge that you have inherited a body-type from your parents that is yours for life? Do you have a nutritional history that may have made a permanent impact on your physique and metabolism? Or have you become a victim of what the educator E.H. Swengel calls "The tyranny of the impossible ideal," and believe that you can, and should, struggle to attain a body shape that is constitutionally beyond your reach? Please remember that a distorted image of one's body is a *common* symptom of anorexia and bulimia. What have responsible friends and family members told you about how you look?

> We will long remember the frustrated conclusion of a bulimic patient we were helping toward an appropriate diagnosis. It was clear that her mother, father, brother, two grandparents, and assorted aunts and uncles were as endomorphic a group as could be found. "My whole freaking family is infested with it!" she exploded.

Coming to terms with our physical destiny can be a humbling experience. Like the boy who always wanted to be a cop but reached adulthood an inch short of the minimum height, many people are desperately anxious to be slender, despite familial tendencies toward robust hips and thighs, which virtually dooms the aspiring ectomorph from the start. Have you become phobic about fat and trained yourself to deny hunger and the pleasure of food in a self-destructive struggle with starvation?

Remember, 98 percent of all patients who lose weight in medically supervised programs eventually regain it again. But the statistics for people who simply resolve, without professional help, to cut down on luxury edibles and who modestly boost their activity levels is far more encouraging. As many as 60 percent of them enjoy long term success in their efforts to reduce.

Perhaps you have simply grown too fond of taking private pleasure in overeating. Or you may have become addicted to the binge-purge cycle after years of trying to rigidly control your appetite without success.

As we have noted earlier, many people contract pathorexia through imposing a regimen of malnutrition on themselves. The STEM program could be misused to create a state of semi-starvation. If that is your goal, you will be abusing yourself and the program.

You may find that weight loss is a legitimate goal, but many, perhaps most, pathorexics will discover that their most important task is to learn to like themselves as heavier-but-healthier than a fashion model. If this is true for you, your task becomes learning to cope with a social environment that values the irrational idea that you can never be too thin.

We believe that many of the consequences of overeating and underexercising can be corrected and that people who carry substantial fat do have some leeway in deciding how much they should weigh. We *do not* believe, however, that basic shapes can be altered.

Unfortunately, we have no formula that prescribes the minimum healthy weight for any one person. We know that pathorexia occurs where weight falls below that individual minimum and that a managable appetite can be restored when weight is regained. But finding that lower boundary to health is a matter for personal discovery. It bears no relationship to fashion and has only a minor relationship to currently available height and weight charts.

Assessing these factors with care (that is, with care for yourself), and reflection will help you decide how much change is healthy for you and how much might further endanger your appetite control. Appendix A has a self-scored evaluation that we use at the University of Connecticut Health Service to help people diagnose their weight and diet status. We urge you to take a few minutes to work through the questionnaire right now and then to take a few more to ponder the significance of your results. Also check your responses to the questionnaire at the end of Chapter 2.

Other excellent sources of information are the books *Fat & Thin* by Anne Scott Beller and *The Dieter's Dilemma* by William Bennett and Joel Gurin (1982). We have listed these and other useful books and articles in Appendix B. Being fully educated about your own problems may well be the toughest piece of research you ever do, but it will be immensely valuable if you can clarify them sufficiently to choose the most appropriate counter-measures.

Even though the general techniques of rehabilitation are similar for all pathorexics, persons with significant physically determined symptoms are quite different from persons with primarily psychological problems. Assuming that one program can treat both disorders will surely result in failure. On the other hand, it is unlikely that anyone with as complex a problem as pathorexia will ever really nail down all the various causes and consequences of their appetite disorder.

It is important, therefore, not to let the search for the perfect diagnosis become an excuse for postponing the start of a plan of therapy. Much effective programming for health can get underway immediately, with modifications and refinements introduced as you become more sophisticated.

Strategy

Careful strategic planning is essential to success. This is as true in personal matters as it is in politics or warfare. The fight against appetite disorder is won by people who recognize how tough a battle they are engaged in. That means reviewing a whole lifestyle, identifying the problem areas, and devising alternative behaviors that will avoid these areas. Ideally, these new activities will actively combat the temptation to abuse food.

Many pathorexics have appetite disorders that are varieties of the temptation to eat too much too often. However, within that generalization are an infinite range of behaviors that make each person unique, with his or her own special problems. If you have identified yourself as a pathorexic, you too have your own patterns of food abuse, with your own ways of allowing them a place in your life.

Most pathorexics are aware of how their eating behavior deviates from healthy practice. They know the times and places where their appetite overcomes their better judgment, or their fear of appetite leads them to take extreme countermeasures. For them, strategic planning means identifying new ways to live that minimize opportunities for those difficulties to arise.

In case you did not catch the message in that last paragraph, let us repeat it. That is right, the strategy needed to overcome a disorder as deeply embedded as pathorexia amounts to nothing less than a new way of living. This can be developed effectively using the STEM program as a guide.

For many people, their revised life is dramatically different from their old one. Changing jobs, roommates, or recreational activities are typical Strategic moves. But that is not always the case.

> Mary is a good example of how changes in lifestyle were accomplished without any visible changes in behavior. She told us, "I've been feeling a lot better lately...I've come to accept my shape...I can't believe it, I never thought I'd be saying that!"
>
> Mary was bulimic when we first saw her. Then she took up dance to compensate for her bingeing. Two years later, she recalled, "My original aim was to stop bingeing, to lose weight, and to have a *perfect* figure. I thought you would help me do that." She paused. "I really feel I've made this progress on my own....Now when I dance, I concentrate on the movement, not on how many calories I'm burning.
>
> "I really don't have the figure for professional work, but I can teach! I'm working on my certificate now. I already teach one class, and I'll be giving another in the fall. And you know what? I'm dating my instructor!"

An example of motivational forces associated with strategy can be drawn from work with drug addiction. While the following represents an exaggerated situation, it serves as a useful analogy. It has been found that drug treatment centers can eliminate all traces of addiction from many heroin users as long as their patients live and work away from home. Their return to the location where they experienced the pain of withdrawal and the relief of pain through drug use often brings back the symptoms they have spent so much time and effort to lose.

There is evidence that the return of those symptoms is partly physiological. There is similar evidence with regard to appetite disorders. Exposure to situations where the symptons were most severe causes a resurgence of unwanted appetite. The saddest aspect of this phenomena is that home, the place of greatest security, may also be the most hazardous situation for the pathorexic.

Your strategies must acknowledge that being in the family kitchen, for example, may arouse a terrible craving to eat and that eating itself does not necessarily quell appetite. Otherwise, your plans will not survive the challenges of daily living.

Although pathorexia may be woven into your life because it is so closely associated with your total environment, much food abuse derives from everyday activities that are consciously distorted to provide opportunities for eating. It is very easy, for instance, to invent little victories during the day for which you can reward yourself with snacks and treats or to make routine social activities occasions for eating.

Our country's vast network of food suppliers (often aided by your family and friends) stand ready to aid and abet you in these petty indulgences. They can provide you with more to eat than you will ever need. And these same commercial interests constantly seek to give you permission to further harm yourself for their benefit.

Only people with normal appetites can resist the countless offers of food that are woven into the fabric of our culture. If you have an urge to eat that exceeds your need to eat, only a campaign that incorporates your whole way of living will effectively and permanently provide the means for a healthy life.

Keeping a safe distance from problem foods usually calls for a reorganization of the pantry and the refrigerator and a reassessment of food purchasing practices. Most people find it helpful, too, to revise their recipes by switching to low-calorie and health-oriented cookbooks.

Such changes, while they are easy to specify, are often difficult to initiate and maintain. Because so many eating behaviors are embedded in tradition and inherited from loved and respected parents and grandparents, you should anticipate a resistance to making these changes, an opposition to continuing them, and frequent temptations to abandon them. It will require your active acceptance of the entire STEM program to make your strategies stick.

Developing a strategy for living is especially difficult for the many pathorexics who have learned to be passive persons. Passivity, like eating, is another quality that is encouraged and rewarded in our society. Many people find that there tends to be fewer problems if they adopt a "go along to get along" attitude in social situations. They excuse their weakness by telling themselves they are being considerate and generous. In fact, they are letting themselves be ruled by other people's decisions—which usually means acting for other people's benefit.

Most passive, dependent people only seem peaceful. Passionate emotions that we all share are hidden from view. The hunger for love, the pressure of anger, and the empty feelings of loneliness are all present inside. These repressed emotions can find symbolic expression in eating behaviors. For example, when the love and attention that agreeableness should earn is not adequately reciprocated, dependent persons may regress to the more primitive comforts provided by cakes, cookies, and other children's treats.

Sometimes, anger inhibited in social and familial situations may find partial release in spasms of vomiting—graphic enactments of the thought, "Such and such person or problem really makes me sick!" or "I have to take things in, digest them and then bring them up later—I can never react spontaneously."

A note here about mental health. Many people who are reluctant to acknowledge emotional problems, such as chronic anxiety or depression, "medicate" themselves by overeating. Such problems are usually readily treated by mental health professionals. If you suspect that you have a tendency to ignore or deny problems or that you substitute one symptom for another, competent counseling may well make the difference between the success and failure of your STEM program's strategy.

To make matters worse, many heavy pathorexics have another hurdle on their path to health—their tendency to move slower and less often than their normal-weight friends. Looked at in a positive light, it could be said such people are efficient organisms, burning fewer calories per hour than the people around them. Unfortunately, their surplus of stored fat means they can become more healthy by becoming more active.

If this is true for you, you may find that mobilizing yourself to burn energy through exercise is one of the hardest changes to make. In the long run, you will discover it to be a rewarding and eventually pleasurable aspect of your new lifestyle. Individuals who have reached a state of stable obesity and who no longer consume more than they expend are well-advised to make increased energy levels their principal method of enhancing health and improving appearance.

Strengthening muscles and improving heart and lung function is the most natural way to raise metabolic rate and trim fat tissue. Aerobic exercises such as walking, dancing, running, swimming, or cycling do not cause increases in lean tissue size, though they may increase muscle density and weight. Instead, they reintroduce you to behaviors your body is designed for but which twentieth century living minimizes or eliminates.

Done in moderation, rediscovering your body's natural functions is a self-reinforcing process that gains momentum continually. Done in excess, exercise becomes an addictive, self-destructive routine that mirrors the victims' beliefs that they do not deserve to feel good about themselves. (many normal and underweight pathorexics are guilty of this).

If you have a tendency towards this kind of excess, you need strategies that set limits on your exercise program so that you maintain fitness and well-being without crowding out more enriching recreational activities.

The exact nature of the exercises that best meet your needs is going to be as individual as the rest of your strategy, but there are some broad guidelines that can be helpful. First, a truly effective program will be one that fits smoothly into your daily routines. If you can actually make it one of your daily responsibilities, so much the better. For people with essentially sedentary occupations, the best opportunity for putting exercise into their schedules is often on the road to work or school.

Walking, running, or cycling to and from work or to and from a strategically parked car can reverse a decline into obesity and subsequent pathorexia by tipping the energy balance into the modest deficit needed to regain health and lose unwanted pounds.

A good example of a person who found a way to include necessary exercise into her life is Lisa, who literally halved her weight from 224 pounds in March to 112 pounds in December, when she first sought treatment from us. She had accomplished this by living solely on a diet product. Lisa looked sick: hollow cheeks, black eye sockets, wispy hair. She was perpetually tired, often dizzy, and was falling victim to a succession of colds and flu.

She came to us because she was scared that she could not stop losing weight and was equally scared about regaining it. It was the second time in eighteen months that she had been this starved.

After we convinced Lisa that only refeeding could save her health, the dam burst on her appetite. We set an initial goal weight as that at which her period returned. When that happened at 145 pounds, she was gaining at the rate of ten pounds a week! She levelled off at 185 pounds, which we discovered was her natural healthy weight and one which she could easily maintain if she got moderate exercise.

Lisa's Strategy was simple. She quit her sedentary job as a cashier, and went back to her old job as a waitress. She also rejoined a bowling league. But before she was able to restore herself to health, Lisa had needed the Educational input that taught her the hazards of attempting to have a body shape that was different from her natural heredity.

Some people who need exercise to maintain health resent the fact that their friends are able to remain essentially inactive without gaining weight. It is important to remember the vast individual differences among us. We need to recognize that a few lucky people are constitutionally well-adapted to an inactive life. Unfortunately, we cannot use their example to justify our own indolence.

Summing up, strategy for most people means making substantial changes in three major areas. The first is rerouting life away from unhealthy food and food related activities while preserving and enhancing normal, pleasurable nutrition. The second is building in a daily opportunity to exercise. The third is seeking insight and solutions for the personal weaknesses that inhibit carrying out the first two decisions.

Good strategies will make changes in ways that add interest and stimulation to your life rather than impose regimens requiring discipline and sacrifice. It is a central concept of the STEM program that you add more than you subtract.

As a final word on Strategy, let us urge you to avoid the trap of allowing a pre-packaged diet plan be your strategy. Neither books, nor organizations, nor experts can specify what you need for you, though many promise to do just that—for a fee.

There is a great temptation for people, faced with the huge problem of pathorexia, to deceive themselves into thinking that they can pay someone else for a solution. Doctors, dietitians, books, and organizations can help, but they cannot cure. Incorporating someone else's plan into your strategy may be a good idea, but making it your whole plan will ensure failure.

Nobody can tell you how to live your life. Overcoming an appetite disorder requires a complex restructuring, and you are the expert, the architect, and the contractor. You need help, but the program and its execution are yours alone.

Tactics

Tactics are the daily implementation of strategic decisions, modified to meet the constant variations that arise in your life. A well-planned strategy creates a health oriented lifestyle. Appropriate tactics reinforce your overall goals in innumerable minor ways that give vitality to your program and blend it into your life.

Your strategy does not merely replace unhealthy activities with healthy ones. It enriches the content of your life by helping you develop autonomy, variety, and sophistication. So tactical approaches emphasize growth, independence, and novelty in more intimate and immediate concerns. Tactics have three purposes: they implement strategy, they combat routine responses, and they stimulate fresh awareness. Put those together and you become a more interesting person.

The daily challenge, if you are pathorexic, is to find ways to keep inappropriate eating out of routine activities and to enlarge your repertoire of healthy behaviors. This is best accomplished by a combination of planned activities and a pre-planned set of responses to unanticipated events.

Planning itself can be broken into two activities: evaluating and scheduling. As you look ahead into the immediate future, you are faced with a variety of activities that you must choose among.

Many of these possibilities are so essential to your well-being that you hardly consider them to be choices: working, washing, eating, sleeping, greeting friends and family, and so on. Other daily events are clearly optional: how you dress and what you do for recreation are typical areas in which you exercise very conscious choices.

In order to engage in your daily round of activities, you must at some point evaluate alternatives, make choices based on your judgement, and then develop a schedule that you follow.

The STEM Program brings that entire process to the forefront of your attention in each of its four parts. Tactics is a matter of evaluating and scheduling possible activities and using their therapeutic value as a criterion for choosing what you will do.

Accepting STEM means accepting responsibility for your life. That acceptance may reach down to the smallest of activities, especially with regard to tactics. It is quite likely that the way you link together the larger portions of your day presents major opportunites for healthy choices that can establish a style for subsequent behaviors.

For example, pathorexics' overactive appetites frequently cause their owners to sneak a snack into breaks in their schedule. As we described in Chapter 8, snacks are more likely to sharpen appetite than to suppress it. Therefore, if eating between meals can be avoided, pathorexia will be eased. The tactical response here may be to seek activities that will undermine the hazardous association between free time and eating.

Alternatives to snacks include recreational walking, shopping, reading a book or newspaper, having conversations, writing letters, knitting or, better yet, doing something for yourself that adds another plus to your day.

Taking responsibility for your life means providing properly for your daily nutritional needs. Nobody has found a better long-term way of doing that than eating balanced meals three or four times a day. All pathorexics resist eating scheduled meals. Anorexics would just as soon not eat; the rest look upon skipping a meal as a way of building up credit that can be used in the next binge.

There is no way you can regain health and still play these games with yourself. Retraining yourself to plan, prepare, and enjoy regular meals is the most important tactical change you can make!

The most effective way that healthy eating can be achieved is through the OA principle "One day at a time." Nobody with an entrenched eating disorder can ever assume that a one-time decision to reform will be powerful enough to last a lifetime. But to hold the line on health from today until tomorrow is a manageable proposition—and the most important single tactic you can employ.

Overeaters and Alcoholics Anonymous have helped millions of people turn their lives around by the use of this simple rule. You can use it today! Then decide tomorrow if you can use it again. Ask yourself, "Can I eat wisely just for today?" Remember, tomorrow remains completely unknown; who knows what you might choose to do then! Make your decision for today alone.

A tactical problem, once you have committed yourself to a day's worth of healthy eating, is coping with unexpected shocks and stresses that you have been accustomed to handling by manipulating your diet. Two questions you can ask yourself at such times are, "Is this worth bingeing over?" or "Is this worth starving over?" Depending on the impulse you are subject to.

If you can make this crucial shift from reaction to reflection in crises, you will be able to master situations that previously overwhelmed you. Notice that the question, "Is this worth bingeing or fasting over?" may at times get a "Yes!" answer!

If disordered eating has been a way of coping with stress for a long time, it is all too likely that the temptation to try the old solution will sometimes be irresistible. That will not mean that your Strategy needs to be changed or that your Tactic of taking one day at a time has been discredited. It simply reminds you that the struggle with pathorexia is difficult and not always won.

Your STEM program uses setbacks as learning opportunities. Ask yourself after a slip, "Was that worth getting sick over?" then seek a more productive way to deal with a similar problem if it should arise in the future. Remember, because you take one day at a time, you start fresh every morning. Some people, at the beginning of their program, make it one hour at a time or even less when they are seriously tempted to backslide.

Like the other three segments of the STEM program, Tactics requires you to shift your decision making from the flawed and obscure processes we described in Chapters 8 and 9 to the rational center of your upper brain—the part of your brain that figured out that you needed to read this book!

Ideally, your awareness of a problem should pave the way to its solution, but in practice we find that that is usually not the case. Even when unconscious forces are made conscious, they are still the same forces pressuring you to act in the same destructive ways. Good tacticians often seek a compromise rather than insist on victory or defeat.

> A recovering pathorexic patient who has learned to stay out of harm's way by visiting her parents' home only briefly and keeping all food out of her own room, said, "I don't like the feeling that I'm not in control, that I can't have food around because if it's there I'll eat it all at once and throw up. But I *do* like the feeling that my life isn't being lived for food anymore."

Better to lose a few battles and win the war than to experience costly victories on minor issues that drain your strength for the long campaign.

> An example of a poor tactic is Dave, who was overweight because his sales job required him to entertain many customers in expensive restaurants.

Dave resolved to end overindulgence once and for all! He made this decision on June 30. The following Friday, July 4th, was the annual family reunion and picnic that Dave traditionally organized and cooked for.

Dave did not handle himself well at the party. He refused to cook anything he believed to be high in calories and boasted about his new lifestyle to his assembled family.

Predictably, they thought Dave was being immature and did not hesitate to say so. In retrospect, Dave agreed with them. He felt foolish and defeated. Within days he was off his diet and back to his old eating patterns.

Many of our clients identify with Dave's dilemma.

Another example where compromise is better than confrontation is the problem of night eating that so often afflicts people who have to study or do similar boring tasks in the evening. For most people, late-evening hunger is triggered by both physical and psychological forces. Falling blood sugar pricks the appetite, and isolation and fatigue lower the resistance to temptation. If earlier in the day a meal has been skipped or even just skimped, the urge to eat will be even more powerful.

The ensuing raid on the refrigerator is physically gratifying but emotionally confusing, as pleasure and planning conflict. Often a psychic numbing results, willpower is suspended, and an extended binge indulged.

Although night eating is usually portrayed as an individual problem, it is often seen as a group phenomenon; for example, when friends get together and spontaneously opt for beer and pizza at midnight—fun while it lasts but deeply regretted the next day.

A variation on this theme, common among pathorexics, is the low-key binge that accompanies irksome responsibilities. Brief periods of work are punctuated by forays for snacks, typically consisting of high-calorie foods and low-calorie drinks. The net intake for an evening may well exceed the caloric totals of the day's three meals, but it is consumed in such small samples that each bite seems insignificant. These transparent self-deceptions are nevertheless enough to sabotage any number of resolutions to reform. Tactically, such occasions are not the time to take a stand against inappropriate eating. It is better to acknowledge them as special weaknesses and to move to minimize the damage.

Plan ahead and have on hand stocks of low-calorie supplies: teas, bouillon, vegetables, and fruit that can be snacked on during the long hours of work. Review both your Strategies and Tactics to see if you can avoid being committed to dull, appetite-provoking activities in the evenings. Opt out of a central role in preparing for feasts. Seek support from friends and family rather than boasting of your new determination to be disciplined.

Other tactical responses are needed to cope with surprise attacks on your appetite. Birthday parties and other celebations require a repertoire of behaviors if you wish to avoid habitual food abuse without losing your friends or your self-respect. This is especially true when alcohol is being served. Only clearly established rules can survive the dulling of good judgment that alcohol induces.

> A specially relevant piece of research warrants mention here. Scientists Peter Herman and Janet Polivy, who have spent many years working on the psychology of eating, found that very many normal-weight people claim that they are very conscious of their desire to overeat and avoid weight gain only through deliberately restrained eating.

> In an experiment, these people were asked to test the flavor of ice creams after drinking small milkshakes. It was found that the more milkshakes their "restrained eaters" were required to consume, the more ice cream they sampled in the flavor test. The researchers were easily able to break the "restrained eaters" resolve to diet by having them drink milkshakes and so precipitate overeating.

> Other people who reported no need to control their eating behaved in the opposite fashion; the more milkshakes they were required to drink, the less ice cream they ate.

A number of useful concepts can be inferred from this simple experiment. First, there are people, lots of them, who effectively maintain normal weight through self-restraint. Second, it is not difficult temporarily to break down that restraint by applying psychological and environmental pressure. Third, and most important, both restraint and failure can co-exist in normal-weight people. In other words, *you do not have to be perfect to succeed*! And finally, it can be concluded that strategies that minimize the likelihood of outside pressure on your appetite and tactics that defend you against those pressures when they arise can make restrained eating a reality in your life.

A final note with regard to alcohol; you should be aware that a significant minority of overeaters are also alcohol abusers, and the two disorders have a good deal in common. Many people with a combined problem attend both Alcoholics Anonymous and Overeaters Anonymous meetings. We are aware of no ongoing treatment programs that can compare with the cost effectiveness or long-term success rate of these two organizations. For people who have lost control of their use of alcohol or whose appetite totally dominates their behavior, a referral to AA or OA is often the first step to regaining control of their lives.

If you believe that you have reached that stage, call AA or OA now. Also, contact by telephone or mail one of the national organizations such as ANAD or NAAS that are dedicated to providing support and therapy for people with appetite disorders. We have listed their addresses and telephone numbers in the Appendix.

Do not expect this book or any other individual self-help program to provide enough insight, motivation, or support to enable you to overcome these disorders alone.

Education

As we have previously emphasized, coming to terms with appetite disorders usually involves acknowledging the need for major changes in living patterns. We have discussed how Strategy and Tactics can help you devise and maintain those changes, but a third essential ingredient for good planning is *good information*—knowing what you are about. The more you know about yourself and your behavior, the better are your chances of making wise choices that can improve your well-being.

While this principle is almost self-evident, it is not that easy to put it into practice in the matter of appetite and eating disorders: not because there is any lack of information, but because there is such a great deal of contradictory views, misinformation, and genuine confusion in both popular and scientific literature.

A consistent effort to be well informed is essential to avoid regression to past practices. There is no way your newly formed Strategies and Tactics will overcome bad habits if they are not properly supported by reliable facts and figures that help you justify choosing the road to health over the rut of illness. Only when you believe that you have learned something about health and about yourself are you mentally equipped to make significant changes in your life.

How do you go about becoming better informed? Very carefully aware from the start that there is more misinformation than good informatic available in both print and broadcast media and in much professionally based material. The suggested readings given at the end of this book provide an introduction to the literature that you will find helpful. Some of the references we cite are most likely to be found in a college or university library. Others can be found at public libraries or in bookstores.

Popular books and magazine articles are much less reliable sources of information. They almost always present overly optimistic assessments and overly narrow viewpoints to be considered responsible. Developments in the field do get reported in the mass media, but researchers' own doubts, questions, and qualifications about their work are often minimized or omitted to keep the stories both exciting and brief.

We have mentioned several books and other publications by name throughout this text, and we urge you to read as many of them as you can find. There are four more publications we feel sure you will find helpful. Two booklets by Lindsay Hall and Leigh Cohn, *Eat Without Fear*, and *Understanding and Overcoming Bulimia*, are short and to the point. A thoughtful book by Kim Chernin, entitled *The Obsession*, deals with the tyranny of thinness. A popular but provocative book for fat people, *Come Out, Come Out, Wherever You Are!*, by Carole Shaw, the editor of the magazine *Big Beautiful Women*, provides wise support to people who are fat. All of these authors have experienced personal struggles with pathorexia.

It is important not to accept anything on trust, but rather put new and interesting information on probation. Test it out and look for confirmation from other sources and from your own experience before incorporating it into your store of knowledge.

Read over Chapters 8 and 9 once more, especially if you skimmed through them the first time. Some of the contents may be a little hard to grasp fully, but you will become familiar with a lot of important scientific research.

As you inquire about psychology and physiology, nutrition and exercise, recreation and pastimes, and so become an informed person, be aware that professional disagreements exist in every area of knowledge. Forewarned is forearmed. Do not let a controversy between experts undermine your own determination to regain your personal health.

A case in point is the dispute over the toxicity of sugar. There are nutritionists who are sure sugar is harmless, while others regard it as

s and indict it for numerous ills and disorders. Chances
ɔmewhere between the two schools of thought. While we
t, prudent pathorexics will be alert to the issue and will
ɛir use of sugar in the light of their own experience with it.

We have ... ɪd that many of our patients are very susceptible to sugar.
One person told us, "When I'm abstinent, I feel fine and act fine, but
when I get into sugar, a tremendous anger erupts within me." Counseling
helped him to recognize that allowing himself to feel the "rush" that
sugar gave him put him in touch with other legitimate but suppressed
"appetites" that he had been striving to ignore because he thought of
them as weaknesses. Although he learned to accept a whole new identity,
sugar remained a hazardous substance for him—but not like it had been
before he sought treatment.

Educating yourself may mean much more than simply reading books and
magazine articles. It can include discovering your personal history by tracking
down medical records. Begin, if you can, by talking with your parents and
your grandparents about your behavior as a child, and try to distinguish
between the reality and the legends about your growth and development.
Concentrate on family customs and values associated with food and eating.

Other contacts with interested people and experts of all kinds can
expand your awareness and understanding of your behavior. Contacts such as
these may forge links between the four parts of the STEM program. Attending
Overeaters Anonymous meetings, for example, would be both a strategic and
a tactical decision, but it would also qualify as an educational experience.
Learning how others cope with their symptoms can be a powerful boost for
your own therapy. The same linkage occurs for strategies that include counseling or psychotherapy, or when a tactical decision to switch from coffee
breaks to reading breaks leads you to new knowledge about health.

Finally, being informed is fun, and sometimes even exciting. Health
maintenance and nutrition are swiftly changing fields where new knowledge is
being generated continually. Obesity and eating disorders are proving to be
extraordinarily complex phenomena, with genetic, organic, and environmental components that were often neglected in the past being studied carefully.

Keeping abreast of advances in understanding of obesity and nutrition
and knowing how personally affected you may be becomes an absorbing
pastime. And, provided you use the information judiciously, it is a valuable
social asset when shared with interested friends.

Monitoring

For many people, the toughest part of their jobs is the paperwork! Keeping accounts is boring and often seems unnecessary. Unfortunately, records are important. Monitoring is a vital component of the STEM program.

Although record keeping sounds dull, when you are moving in the right direction, it becomes a continuing success story, and that is not dull at all! Your diary of progress is a powerful inducement to further progress. The more closely you monitor your behavior, the greater is your incentive to make that behavior rewarding and to improve on past performance.

There is a second and more important reason for monitoring your behavior when you combat pathorexia: it is a great help in raising your conscious awareness of what you are doing. The central disorder in pathorexia is that your instincts no longer correspond with your needs—what you want to do makes you ill. It therefore becomes essential that you take charge of your instincts and that you accept more responsibility for your behavior. Like administrators everywhere, that means you increase the paperwork.

So what is meant by monitoring? There are two major processes involved: recording what you intend to do and recording what you have done and how you feel about your performance. People with severe eating disorders, when they are not blocking out all their feelings about food, often feel guilty and upset about everything that goes into their mouths. Because they are so prone to abuse food, they perceive all eating as wrong.

A safe way out of this dilemma is a technique pioneered to Overeaters Anonymous in which an appropriate selection and quantity of food is *committed* at the beginning of the day. The recovering overeater is then free to enjoy thoroughly three of four guilt-free meals. All other foodstuffs are off limits—no point in even thinking about them. Research studies have shown that the principle is a good one.

Planning ahead and specifying precisely what you regard as acceptable behavior greatly enhances the likelihood of your staying within those healthy limits. It is important when you do this that you plan for an adequate and nutritionally complete menu. If you plan too spare a menu for the day, there will come a moment of self-pity with a spasm of unscheduled overeating.

This principle applies to more than just eating. Your exercises or studies are far more likely to be completed if they are comfortably within your abilities and scheduled ahead of time. Good management requires good planning, so set healthy, attainable goals.

In the journal that develops from monitoring your progress, there can be space for notes and comments about your Strategy and Tactics. Here is where you commit to writing what you want to accomplish, the long term plans that can achieve those goals, and the dozens of tricks and techniques that can help on a daily basis.

Also record any other information that may be specially pertinent for you: facts and statistics about nutrition and health, personal statistics. Even a wish list of desirable rewards and treats you can celebrate with. A working journal soon takes on a life of its own. It becomes the natural place to file phone numbers, friends' birthdays, and anything else you need to have at your fingertips.

As you build up a store of information and become accustomed to adding to and drawing from your journal, you enormously reinforce the rational powers of your brain, because record keeping is a rational process.

Do not assume or be concerned that Monitoring might transform you into a cold, logical being, as just the reverse is more likely to occur. You will become emotionally freer, more relaxed, and more able to enjoy the good things in life as you lose the nagging fear that you are an inept, undisciplined failure at life's important tasks.

Having a plan and sticking to it gives you confidence in yourself, and having a journal in which to confide your hopes, apprehensions, successes, and disappointments helps you validate your emotions and accept them for what they are—the color and spice of your life, a daily reminder of your unique nature.

Almost as important as looking ahead is keeping track of what is actually happening to you. In retrospect this will be the enjoyable part of Monitoring. A "mood and food" diary, recording everything that makes a day notable, quickly becomes a fascinating account of progress. Although, for a pathorexic person, changes in eating behaviors will be emphasized in the record, a journal gains depth and character and insight only when emotional matters are included.

Self-knowledge requires self-examination and reflection. Confiding regularly in a diary is one of the better ways to achieve this. Inevitably, the issues that give you the most trouble get referred to repeatedly. As the record grows, it becomes harder to ignore or excuse patterns of failure, and it becomes easier to discover how those patterns operate. The relationships between your environment, your appetites, your emotions, and your behaviors are clarified. With this knowledge, you can take steps toward a more self-directed, autonomous lifestyle, no longer seeing yourself as a victim of circumstance.

A journal becomes an effective tool only when it is used. That means you need frequently to read over what you have written to compare the present with the past. This permits you to engage in a dialogue with yourself about the most important matters in your life. When your journal includes candid, unvarnished, and unedited opinions about your strengths (be sure not to forget these) and weaknesses, you greatly increase your awareness of yourself.

If you find yourself continuing to behave in ways that mystify and depress you, despite this feedback, think about professional counseling as a means of greater insight and control. Working with a psychotherapist on these problems will enable you to receive objective feedback. Together, you will be able to devise a more powerful STEM program.

Because your journal is the active center of your entire STEM program, it is important that you treat it with respect. The more you invest in your journal, the better it will serve you. Begin by purchasing a quality hardcover journal. Something that will look good and will wear well. After all, it is going to be Volume I of a very important autobiography! The design, size and number of pages can reflect your personal preference, but do not skimp on quality—your story is too valuable to be committed to a junky notebook.

To conclude this chapter, we want to emphasize a theme we have sounded throughout this book. We want to remind you that pathorexia is a stubborn, hard-to-correct disorder, but that its progress can be halted and held in remission through a far-reaching revision of customary behaviors.

Arresting pathorexia will change your life, but you must change your life to arrest pathorexia. Because this is so, it is essential to think of the STEM program as a continuing project that has neither a timetable nor a termination.

Keep in mind that nothing worthwhile is accomplished without error. Little worth doing is done right the first time. Testing your program by finding out what strategies, tactics, and record keeping methods do not work for you is part of the process of discovering what *does* work.

Recognizing the importance of trial-and-error in forming your program is a giant step toward undermining the perfectionism so prevalent among pathorexics. Work your program a step at a time, gathering strength and confidence as you go. But anticipate setbacks, and refuse to be discouraged simply because you temporarily slip back into an all too familiar rut.

One final word: *share your program.* Look for a person or persons who will endorse your commitments and support your efforts, especially when you experience failure. If you feel that you cannot confide in a friend or cannot afford a therapist, yet you need more support, call Overeaters Anonymous.

OA has over twenty years of experience working with the symptoms of pathorexia, It's members have a lot of respect for the disease and a record of achievement that gives hope to even the most discouraged person. Restored by the support of understanding people, you can return to your program once more, gain another day of healthy behavior, and a further increment of self-respect.

11
therapeutic metaphor*
images for growth

"He is there when I awaken
Makes his presence known
Speaks to me alone
that which must never be uttered aloud
I succumb to no other."

There are many approaches to the treatment of obesity and appetite disorders. This chapter introduces a relatively new one that can serve as an aid to the STEM program. Problems with multiple causes require a variety of approaches in order to create effective change. A technique called *Therapeutic Metaphor* may be useful to you or your therapist in assisting you to lose weight, maintain weight loss, or uncover feelings that will help in recovering from appetite disorders. Basically metaphors may be used:

1. to uncover underlying feelings;
2. to reveal hidden solutions;
3. to create an aversion to undesirable but tempting foods;

*Much of this chapter is based on Adams, Cynthia, and Joan Chadbourne, "Therapeutic Metaphor: An Approach to Weight Control," *Journal of the American Personnel and Guidance Assoc.*, 60, (April 1982), 510. It is reprinted by permission of the publisher.

4. to provide a person with a new self concept; and
5. to increase compliance with treatment techniques.

While this chapter will not teach you HOW to write a metaphor, it will provide a rationale for the development and use of metaphors as a therapeutic technique, give actual case examples, and provide sample metaphors that we have used.

Definition and Demonstration

Generally, a metaphor is "a figure of speech in which one thing is likened to another....it is an implied comparison, in which a word or phrase ordinarily and primarily used for one thing is applied to another" (e.g., "screaming headlines," "all the world's a stage"), to use the definition in Webster's dictionary.

A therapeutic metaphor is a use of this figure of speech in a way that lets victims of appetite disorders recognize themselves, their problems, and possible new alternatives, in a non-confrontive and non-threatening way. This is especially helpful in dealing with feelings, like anger, that many people are taught not to express.

The following is an example used to help a victim see outside of her "trap" to discover that choices exist. Here, one of the authors employed a metaphor as a method of sharing information symbolically that might not have been accepted directly.

When her mother left, the little pony sulked in her stall. She put her head down low and only looked at the floor. She spent days just eating and sulking, eating and sulking, never looking outside her window. She didn't see the sun shining, hear the birds singing, or feel the warmth all around her. She didn't see the little butterfly that rested on her window waiting to play—her head was down and all she knew was the pleasure of grain.

Then one day the farmer gently led the pony outside. At first she could not perceive the beauty all around her, but soon she was frolicking and rolling in the tall grass. Other ponies soon came to play. Life had warmth and fun.

The "little pony" is a metaphor for the victim. Describing her, in this instance, as little is actually symbolic of a sense of helplessness rather than a reference to physical size. The reference to the "mother" leaving is used to indicate a loss in *this* victim's life that seems to have caused the overeating.

Choices for the victim, other than "eating and sulking," were shown to exist by mentioning "the sun shining," "the birds singing," "the little butterfly," and "the feeling of warmth." The metaphor ended with the victim keeping her head down, knowing only the "pleasure of grain." But to demonstrate the alternatives, we had the farmer gently lead the pony outside. Here the farmer symbolizes the helping professional assisting the victim in exploring healthy alternatives.

It should be evident from reading the above description that therapeutic metaphors must be tailored to the individual. Thus, in this example, we would have to understand what in the victim's life related to the overeating (in this case it was personal loss) and further decide on a preferred course of action (alternative coping behaviors) for the patient before designing the metaphor.

This therapeutic metaphor is intended to convey, subtly and symbolically the fact that there are better options all around, that she need only lift up her head to see that her life can be different. Symbolism connects at an emotional level when direct confrontation raises defences. It assists the victim in changing at an unconcious as well as conscious level because it is less threatening. This particular example is best used in a therapeutic environment. However, examples for self-help appear later in this chapter.

Therapeutic Metaphor as a Treatment for Appetite Disorder

This section will explore the further uses of therapeutic metaphor as a means of promoting recovery from appetite disorders. A crucial factor here will be the determination of those specific factors that contributed both to the development of the problem and the failure of previous treatment programs. How the metaphor is designed and what course of action it proposes depends upon what we discover the about the patient's personal history.

Five descriptions are used to demonstrate the application of the therapeutic metaphor to treatment of pathorexia. The first four are geared toward use by health professionals; the fifth sample may be useful as a self-help technique. Certainly, there are additonal possibilities not discussed here.

First we will view the therapeutic metaphor as a means of accessing some of the victim's history around fat, for fat often has symbolic meaning. We have allowed victims to describe themselves symbolically through metaphor. This has often revealed important information. In the example that follows, we simply asked Anne to name the food that was most like her.

> She said: "I am a huge stuffed pepper."
> Counselor: "Can you explain that further?"
> Anne: "Yes, I'm huge and stuffed because I'm hot, angry—the stuffing keeps me cool."

As we explored this anger further, it appeared that Anne was unable to express her anger before except by flaunting her fatness. Her metaphor revealed this *hidden* anger. Treatment proceeded by focusing on the need to express this anger. Until she learned to deal with the anger, no diet was going to succeed.

A second application of the metaphor for appetite disorder is its use as a supplement to other treatment. A client at our clinic reported that she could control her overeating if she could manage to resist canned foods.

The client was encouraged to enter a state of deep relaxation and then *imagine* what might make her stop eating canned foods. She came upon the idea of maggots wriggling inside a can of tuna fish. She held this image, explored it, and developed it so that it became more of an experience than a fantasy. Whenever temptation arose she responded by inducing her metaphor. Thus, outside of direct therapy she was able to use the technique. Subsequently, she ceased eating canned foods.

Metaphors can also be used to assist people who deny the reality of their own bulk: clients who may have been referred by physicians for help in getting rid of dangerous pounds, or who are seeking assistance to "please" someone else, but who do not *really* wish to lose weight. Another form of this denial is those individuals who pretend to diet but do not. (Certainly there are individuals who cannot lose weight—here, however, we refer to those who do not lose, but claim they are "trying.")

These persons are excellent candidates for a therapeutic metaphor. Information about appropriate dietary intakes or behavioral programs is generally ignored. However, a metaphoric anecdote that provides the appropriate information is much more likely to lead them to successful compliance. The case of a 63-year-old man who "wasn't sure if he really wanted to diet" illustrates the concept.

There once was a man who walked high wires all his life. But he had always used a net because he wanted to protect himself. Well, even walking high wires can get boring after enough years have passed. So this man decided to try a very high wire *without* a net. Now, his wife didn't like this idea. She thought he was too old to take such a chance. What did he need to prove, anyway? But the man was determined. He was determined to walk the wire for himself and for the world. So he went to see an engineer. And the engineer gave him a special balancing stick with precise instructions, so he knew just how to use that stick to make the walk along the high wire without a net.

(1) In this metaphor, we have used the net to represent a form of protection. Fat metaphorically protects the patient. It is symbolized by the net. (2) Wanting to walk the wire without a net represents the individual's desire for change, although there is risk involved. (3) The reaction of his wife is a typical sabotage phenomenon that occurs in dieters' families. (4) The engineer is the dietitian, educator, or counselor. The balancing stick and instructions on how to use it represent dietary knowledge given to the client.

The therapeutic metaphor may be used to prepare the individual's self concept for the change in body size that follows weight change. Victims are asked to picture themselves as they will appear after appropriate weight gain or loss; they visualize themselves with "normal" figures, with the same attributes as other healthy people in their families.

Finally, therapeutic metaphors can be used almost hypnotically, in a relaxing manner, to redirect thoughts for a positive approach to controlling eating. The two metaphors that follow are examples of this which can be used by the reader alone or with the help of a friend or therapist.

This one helps anorexia victims overcome their fear of eating.

YOUR FAVORITE FRUIT
What is your favorite fruit?

Can you picture the tree that bears this fruit? Picture the tree as its buds fill out, then open. Can you see it in full bloom and enjoy the colors and the smell of the blossoms in the wind? Now imagine a gentle rain washing away the petals after the bees have visited. Then the sun shines down. Warm and strong. Soon the fruit is visible and at last ripened by the sun.

Picture yourself as you walk toward the tree. You are carrying a basket. Fill the basket with the delightful fruit. Now sit in the shade and begin to eat your harvest. Admire the beauty of the fruit, the texture of the skin. Now bite into the fruit, feel its coolness in your mouth, let the juices run down your chin, smell the delicious fruit flavor. It is lush and its goodness is good for you.

You may eat it whenever you want.

In contrast, the next metaphor helps correct the compulsive eater's fears.

HUNGER IS YOUR FRIEND

I want you to close your eyes and relax. Take a few deep breaths and relax further. Now that you are feeling very comfortable and very relaxed, I want you to imagine that you have a magic friend who can help you lose weight if you will allow him or her to. This friend can help you lose weight faster than a low-calorie meal, faster even than exercise. This friend is Hunger.

I want you to picture yourself and describe him or her to me in detail. Now I want you to describe all the ways Hunger can help you lose weight.

The first thing we must understand is that Hunger, like any friend, should be greeted happily and should be accepted with joy, not rejected. You know when Hunger comes to visit that you are actually losing weight right that minute. Hunger brings you the gift of *knowing* that the changes you want are actually taking place.

If you can accept Hunger and not frighten him or her away by rushing to eat something, you can then allow the visit to last long enough to give your body wonderful favors. You can picture Hunger warming and then melting away your *ugliest* fat while he or she visits, taking away your least-desired inches. The service of a true friend.

When Hunger leaves for a few hours, you know what to do to prepare for his or her return and can plan for it and rejoice when you are together again.

Hunger is your friend.

Therapeutic Metaphor and Weight Maintenance

People who lose weight after a long period of obesity may not see themselves as normal unless they have been prepared in advance for the change. Even when hundreds of pounds have been shed, previously obese individuals are apt to see themselves as heavy, as did those people who were always fat, were never chosen to be on sports teams, were never asked to dance in high school, never ran fast, and have no experience of certain kinds of athletic and physical movements.

The Rockefeller Institute studied this phenomenon in a group of formerly superobese patients. They reported persistent feelings of largeness, surprise when someone would or could sit down next to them on a bus, and surprise at any spontaneous, favorable reaction to them such as a whistle or a compliment from a stranger.

Through the use of metaphors, whole new pasts can be created to help such people. Here is an example we used with one person:

> "I'm walking toward school, the sun is out, and I see other kids coming along the sidewalks on their way to school, too. Some kids are riding bikes and some are running. I'm feeling really free and light, so I skip for awhile. Pretty soon, my friend Jill catches up to me and soon we're singing and laughing and skipping. I have on a new green outfit made out of thin material that floats in the air as I move. I can feel the air on my face and I know I can run so fast that nobody will catch me.
>
> "Now we get to school, and I'm not even out of breath. I have so much energy. People are smiling at me and asking me my name and what street I live on. I'm just smiling back. Then the teacher talks to us about how she expects us to behave and who uses which side of the coat room.
>
> "Finally, it's recess, and I get picked to be captain of the kickball team!"

You do not need to be especially creative to superimpose a "new way" over often harsh memories. Regular daydreaming over an extended period of time can help you develop a rich and complete past that affords you understanding and poise in the present. The new self concept thus better maintains the *new* body.

Via the metaphor, you may gain experience that was previously lost to you. You face the world with a different self, without the old feelings of vulnerability or defensiveness. You may even allow this *new person* to be typically human and not have to make ALL of life's promises come true.

ARLENE

Arlene was a 30-year-old woman when she came for therapy after 20 years of bulimic behavior. For many of those years, she believed herself to be healthy because she was convinced that fasting, vegetarianism, and bran were sacred. In many ways, she was a flower child of the 1960s, lost in a time warp.

At times, when Arlene was in touch with her disorders, both physically and mentally, she had sought the help of a variety of "experts." Unfortunately, all failed to diagnose her correctly and treated her with an array of ineffective techniques ranging from diets to fad psychotherapies. By the time we told her there was a name for her disorder and that she wasn't alone with her problem, she was severely depressed, bordering on suicide, and limited in her ability to function at her job.

A typical day for Arlene involved a breakfast of bran, yeast, yogurt, and fruit followed by an enema. She would drag herself to work in order to survive financially, but she felt unrewarded and demeaned by the job itself. Frequently working on the road, she would stop at convenience stores to indulge in sweets. The end of the day would find her depressed, angry with herself, and hiding at home, sometimes with the blinds drawn. She would literally pray that no one would drop in and felt safest when the phone was disconnected.

There were many things about which Arlene was angry: her family for making her believe she was a "golden child" when the rest of the world did not respond to her that way; her Dad for always being sick with a heart condition; and herself for being so trapped. But she held all this anger in and could only release it into the toilet bowl.

Arlene was finally able to acknowledge her anger and release it verbally when she metaphorically saw her illness as a Dragon, a Dragon that controlled her life and was everywhere waiting to "get her" until she fought back. She wrote the following poem, and we worked on slaying the Dragon. Within a few weeks, she was able to toss out her enema bag and is now a recovering pathorexic.

THE DRAGON

He is there when I awaken
Makes his presence known
Speaks to me alone
that which must never be uttered aloud
I succumb to no other

Silent pool in wait
Unnoticed in darkness
Erupts in fire never emptying
Yet ever contained
Senses rage, bleed, fail
offering pain for pain
More easily borne
(once upon a time)

Seeking escape in
narrowing spaces
intimately bound
living only in each other

Pray to strength
to endure
to let be and let go
to breathe to share
to surrender anew

21 March 1982

appendix A
self-evaluation exercise

This appendix includes a self-evaluation tool that we use at the University of Connecticut Health Service. *Calorie Counters are Losers* was prepared for patients consulting the University Nutritionist, Maryann Ludwig. We have found it to be useful and thought provoking. It is especially helpful for people who are planning a STEM program.

Calorie Counters Are Losers*

We live in a culture preoccupied with being slim. Most people think that the fatter you are, the more—and more carelessly—you've been eating, and the skinnier you are, the less you've been eating, the more self control you have. This is not always true. This line of thinking leads to poor eating habits, guilt, unhappiness, and even discrimination against fat people.

The truth is, every body is different. Most people fall into three main categories. To find out what category your body is in, take the following quiz:

*Written by Maryann Ludwig, M.S., R.D., and Vivian Mayer. Used with permission. Ms. Mayer is active in the fat liberation movement.

1. How long have you considered yourself "too fat"?

    A. only in the last year
    B. since puberty
    C. since early childhood

2. What is the most "overweight" you have ever been?

    A. 5-10 lbs.
    B. 10-25 lbs.
    C. 25-50 lbs.
    D. over 50 lbs.

3. How often have you been within 5 lbs. of the weight you would like to weigh?

    A. until recently
    B. occasionally after dieting
    C. rarely, even after dieting
    D. never

4. How many other people in your biological family are fat?

    A. no one else
    B. one parent and/or a sibling
    C. both parents
    D. one or more parents and siblings

5. Which of the statements below best describes the kind of eating behavior you worry most about and want to change?

    A. when my friends are eating snacks, I can't resist joining them
    B. I frequently eat large meals
    C. I nibble constantly between meals
    D. I stay on a diet for a few days or weeks but then go on an uncontrolled food binge.

6. How often in the past 5 years have you tried to lose weight?

    A. never
    B. once
    C. several times
    D. I'm always trying to lose weight

Now evaluate your score. The number of points for each response is at the intersection of the rows and columns corresponding to each response. Add the total score. Then identify which group you probably belong to. (If you score very near the border between groups, you should read the information pertaining to both groups.)

SCORING	A	B	C	D
7	1	2	4	5
8	1	3	4	4
9	1	2	4	5
10	1	2	3	-

Basically Slim (total score 6-12) You have been slim or of average weight most of your life. A recent change in your lifestyle has resulted in less physical exercise and/or more opportunities to eat high-calorie foods than before. You may have gained 10 lbs. and want to "get back in shape."

Chronic Dieters (total score 13-17) You've never been so fat as to have to buy your clothes in special stores. But those few *extra* pounds keep nagging at you. Lately you may be finding it harder and harder to keep them off.

Chronic Dieters Plus (total score 18 or greater) Unless you stick to a low calorie diet, you tend to be fat. You may have been fat since early childhood, or since adolescence. You may have tried many times to lose weight. Each attempt ultimately failed, and left you fatter than ever.

For Everyone

The special needs of each group will be discussed later. First, here are some general suggestions that apply to everyone.

1. A well-balanced diet, sufficient in calories, high in fresh produce and low in refined sugar, processed food, etc, is good for nearly everyone. There should be no "forbidden foods." You should never deliberately keep yourself hungry.

2. Supply yourself with minimally processed foods to snack on: whole grain breads and muffins, fresh fruit and vegetables.

3. Make room in your life for non-food oriented activities that you enjoy.

4. Exercise should be something you enjoy. If you don't enjoy your present form of exercise, try something else.

5. Avoid artificial sweeteners and special diet foods. These foods interfere with your natural appetite regulating system.

6. Fatness is not a sure sign of overeating. Careful studies have shown that the calorie intakes of fat and slim people fall within the same range.

7. Dieting may make you temporarily slimmer, but it has some consequences that tend to make you fatter in the long run: A. the longer you go with insufficient calories, the stronger the urge to binge, especially on sugary foods; B. the longer you go with insufficient calories, the more efficient your metabolism becomes. Ultimately you may get as many calories out of an apple as a typical non-dieter gets out of a piece of apple pie. The result? Every time you stop dieting you gain back more than you lose.

8. We live in a culture with a heavy investment—both financially and emotionally—in the idea that the average mature body is "too fat." Hence you feel real pain when you look in the mirror. Given the types of food propaganda we face in our society, it is helpful to be conscious of how we eat, and make deliberate choices. It is not helpful to be preoccupied with food.

You may not have been told these things before, but that is because people only told you things that would keep you trying to lose weight.

IF YOU SCORED BASICALLY SLIM:

1. For one week, substitute a piece of fresh fruit for your ordinary sweet snacks and desserts. Have fresh fruits and vegetables on hand for snacking.

2. Eat slowly, eat the main course, and do not limit yourself solely to salads and vegetables at meal times. Carbohydrates and proteins in moderate quantities are necessary for optimal health.

3. Eat three meals daily at regualr times. Structure your meals so there is a beginning and an end.

4. If you cook for yourself, decrease amounts of fat in food being cooked but don't eliminate fat altogether, as it adds nutrition and tends to make people feel "full."

5. A few extra pounds gained by "careless eating" should come off easily but gradually if you don't try to force them. But if these small changes don't make you slimmer, relax. It is natural to gain a little weight as one matures. Recent evidence suggests that a little "extra" weight (compared with current fashion) actually improves your health.

IF YOU SCORED CHRONIC DIETER OR CHRONIC DIETER PLUS:

These groups are very similar. People who score in these groups have been worrying about their weight for a long time. The main difference is the amount of weight they've been worrying about.

If you are a chronic dieter, regardless of your size, you have probably seen the suggestions that were made for Group 1 many times. You don't need them now. In fact, your nutrition and metabolism may be changed from frequent dieting so that suggestions that involve eating less are irrelevant or even harmful to you.

IF YOUR SCORE WAS AROUND 13-17:

If you think you're in real danger of becoming very fat, you're right! Only the danger comes from where you least expect it. Not from the extra piece of cake, but from the dieting.

To understand this, go back to the section "For Everyone" and reread points 6, 7, & 8. Whatever you do about your weight, you must take these facts into account.

IF YOU SCORED OVER 17:

Guilt—undeserved—may be your biggest problem. Being fat is not a "fault." Even if you think of yourself as a "compulsive eater," such problems are not a "fault." In fact, similar eating behaviors have been created in laboratory animals by keeping them on low calorie diets.

The same rules of good nutrition that apply to slim people apply to you. You should not short-change yourself of any nutrients, including calories.

Has Worrying About Your Weight
Affected Your Nutrition and Self-Respect?

Please take the following quiz:

7. How do you feel when you eat something extra, like a dessert or high calorie snack, that you were not planning to eat?

  A. I enjoy it
  B. I enjoy it, with regrets
  C. I enjoy it, but feel very guilty and angry at myself afterwards
  D. I feel out of control and unreal——

8. Which of the statements below best describes the way you feel about the exercise or active sport you engage in (or if you don't do any, how you feel when people tell you you should)?

  A. I do it for fun
  B. I get tired of it, but keep it up for health reasons
  C. My major reason is to stay slim or to lose weight
  D. I feel forced to exercise because my body embarrasses me——

9. Which of the statements below best describes the pattern of your calorie intake?

  A. almost the same from day to day
  B. once in a while I overeat, but I make up for it carefully
  C. periods of dieting that may last for days or weeks, then periods of bingeing on food
  D. I overeat, then make myself vomit or take laxatives to stay slim——

10. Have you ever received psychological counseling to help you lose weight?

  A. no
  B. no, but I thought about it
  C. yes ——

QUESTIONS	A	B	C	D
1	1	2	3	-
2	1	2	3	5
3	1	3	4	4
4	1	3	4	5
5	1	1	2	4
6	1	1	2	2

If you scored near or above 11, you may be losing a lot more than weight. Information in this book can help you combat narrow-minded social attitudes. But please keep in mind that yours is a societal problem, not just a "personal problem."

To Help You Start Winning

1. There are a lot of other people who have had the same struggles with eating and weight. Ask your local counseling center to help you organize fat consciousness raising groups that are separate from weight loss groups. Such groups provide positive, constructive insights and solutions.

2. It may be difficult for you to reestablish a sense of nutritional balance. You may lose weight or gain weight. Be patient with yourself. You're allowed to make mistakes.

3. Celery and other raw vegetables are excellent munchies for well-fed people, but they are no substitutes for adequate calories. Try fruit, cheese, nuts, etc., especially if you have been on a low-calorie diet for a long time.

4. As you add to your wardrobe, buy new clothes with an emphasis on comfort and ease of movement.

5. Seek out people and activities that reinforce your sense of your own intelligence, your good personality, or your other abilities. You are more than a body to be judged by other people.

YOUR OPTIONS:

To continue the losing struggle

—OR—

To learn respect and live in your body whether or not
its natural size is fashionable.

THE WINNER'S BOX

There's a place for everyone here no matter what your
size.

A balanced diet, sufficient calories, and exercise you
enjoy
are winning strategies for nutritional balance, health, and
self-confidence.

---

appendix B
additional sources
of assistance

Many local and at least four national organizations exist to help victims of pathorexia. If you live in an urban or suburban area, you can almost surely find support and therapy through listings in your telephone book. Community Mental Health Centers can be located under Social Service Organizations in the Yellow Pages. Most University Health Services have enough experience with appetite disorders to enable them to refer you for help even if you are not a student. State Mental Health Associations often have listings of qualified therapists.

The two major self-help organizations, Overeaters Anonymous (OA) and Alcoholics Anonymous (AA) are listed in most larger telephone directories, or you can find them by calling Directory Information for the nearest large city near your home. They welcome initial inquiries by telephone and will help you make arrangements to attend a meeting by providing a sponsor and often a ride if you need one. Their national headquarters are listed below.

The following national organizations will also put you in touch with local sources of support.

The American Anorexia/Bulimia Association
(formerly The American Anorexia Nervosa Association)
133 Cedar Lane
Teaneck, New Jersey 07666
Telephone (201) 836–1800

The National Anorexia Aid Society
P.O. Box 29461
Columbus, Ohio 43216
Telephone (614) 846–6810

**The National Association of Anorexia Nervosa
and Associated Disorders**
P.O. Box 271
Highland Park, Illinois 60035
Telephone (312) 831–3438

The National Association to Aid Fat Americans, Inc.
P.O. Box 43
Bellerose, New York 11426
Telephone (516) 352–3120

Overeaters Anonymous
3730 Motor Avenue
Los Angeles, California 90034

Alcoholics Anonymous
P.O. Box 459
Grand Central Station
New York, New York 10017

American Society of Bariatric Physicians
333 West Hampden Avenue # 307
Englewood, Colorado 80110

suggested readings

Adams, Cynthia H., and Paul Haskew, "A Perspective on Appetite Disorder," *American Pharmacy* (periodical), Vol. NS22, No. 11, p. 51, November 1982.

Beller, Anne Scott, *Fat and Thin: A Natural History of Obesity,* New York: Farrar Straus & Giroux, Inc., 1976.

Bennett, William and Joel Gurin, *The Dieter's Dilemma,* New York: Basic Books, Inc., 1982.

Boskind-White, Marlene and William C. White, *Bulimarexia: The Binge/Purge Cycle,* New York: W.W. Norton, 1983.

Bray, George, (Ed.)., *Obesity in America,* Washington, DC: Department of Health, Education, and Welfare Publication, 1979.

Bruch, Hilde, *Eating Disorders,* New York: Basic Books, Inc., 1973

———, *The Golden Cage: The Enigma of Anorexia Nervosa,* Cambridge, MA: Harvard Press, 1978.

Cauwels, Janice M., *Bulimia: The Binge-Purge Compulsion,* Garden City, NY: Doubleday and Company, Ltd., 1983.

Chernin, Kim, *The Obsession: Reflections on the Tyranny of Slenderness,* New York: Harper and Row, 1981.

Goldman, William, *Tinsel*, New York: Bellaconte Press, 1979.

Hall, Lindsey and Leigh Cohn, *Eat Without Fear* (booklet), Santa Barbara, CA: Gurze Press, 1980.

———, *Understanding and Overcoming Bulimia* (booklet), Santa Barbara, CA: Gurze Press, 1982.

Kinoy, Barbara P., (Ed.), *"When Will We Laugh Again": Living and Dealing With Anorexia and Bulimia*, New York: Columbia University Press, 1984.

Levenkron, Steven, *The Best Little Girl in the World*, New York: Warner Books, 1979.

———, *Treating and Overcoming Anorexia Nervosa*, New York: Scribner's Sons, 1982.

Lindner, R.M, *The 50 Minute Hour*, New York: Rhinehart, 1961.

Mayer, J., *Overweight—Causes, Cost and Control*, Englewood Cliffs, NJ: Prentice-Hall, Inc., 1969.

Orbach, S., *Fat is a Feminist Issue*, New York: Berkley Publishing Corp., 1979.

Polivy, Janet and C. Peter Herman, *Breaking the Diet Habit: The Natural Weight Alternative*, New York: Basic books, Inc., 1983.

Schoenafielder, Lisa and Barb Weiser (Eds.) *Shadow on a Tightrope: Writings by Women on Fat Oppression*, Iowa City, Iowa: Aunt Lute Book Company, 1983.

Shaw, Carole, (Ed.), *Big Beautiful Women* (periodical), Encino, CA, 91316

Shaw, Carole, and Hank Nuwer, *Come Out, Come Out, Wherever You Are!*, Los Angeles: American R.R. Publishing Co., 1982.

Sheldon, William H., *Atlas of Men*, New York: Harper and Bros., 1954.

———, *The Varieties of Temperament*, New York: Harper, 1942.

Stunkard, Albert S., *Obesity*, Philadelphia: Saunders, 1980.

———, *The Pain of Obesity*, Palo Alto, CA: Bull Publishing Co., 1980.

index

A

[